MEDITERRANEAN
DIET COOKBOOK FOR BEGINNERS:

Table Of Contents

Introduction

People from the Mediterranean countries are known to live longer and healthier lives compared to most Americans. There are many reasons for that, but the main one is the difference in lifestyles and diets. Not that the people around the Mediterranean are spared from evil diseases such as cancer or heart failures, but the number of such illnesses is significantly lower.

When you hear about the Mediterranean, the first thing that comes to your mind is the great food, delicious wine, sunshine, lovely islands, and people who look utterly content.

There is no secret; these people tend to eat lots of fresh fruits and vegetables. Some of the best Mediterranean meals contain nothing but vegetables and olive oil.

So, when your diet is mainly based on eating fruits, vegetables, fish, nuts, and healthy oils, it is no wonder that your body is fit and you are not as prone to diseases such as diabetes and cancer.

The Mediterranean diet is not a new thing. People living around the Mediterranean Sea (Balkans, Italy, Spain, Turkey, etc.) were always consuming local foods. This area around the largest sea in the world is sun-kissed for more than three hundred days a year; no wonder here you can find some of the freshest and most delicious fruits and vegetables, aromatic spices, delicious wines and fresh juices, light meals that will satisfy your taste buds and keep you full for a long time.

The popularity of this diet rose in the sixties when Mediterranean restaurants found their way to the rest of the world.

The secret lies in the fact that the Mediterranean Diet is focused on whole-grain foods, healthy fats (olive oil, nuts, fish), fruits, vegetables, and very small amounts of red meat.

But, what most people don't know about this diet is the fact that it encourages people to cook and eat their meals with their families. Naturally, for an even better effect, the Mediterranean Diet is twice as better when you involve physical activity.

People who live around the Mediterranean are known hedonists; they love good food and good drinks, don't rush their meals and dedicate their attention to the food they eat. But, besides the good food, they are not lazy and would gladly use their bike or walk from one place to another.

Every meal in this diet is equally important, and you are not advised to starve to see visible results on your body.

This diet requires you to start the day with a light breakfast, such as oatmeal. Naturally, a light breakfast won't keep you full for a long time; this is why the Mediterranean Diet suggests a piece of fruit as a snack between breakfast and lunch.

Lunch usually includes a delicious salad that contains lots of vegetables mixed with cheese or nuts, while the dinner is reserved for a more substantial dish (fish, vegetables, cuscus, etc.).

The main reason for that is because carbs are not bad per se; when mixed with the right amount of healthy fats (fish and other seafood), vegetables and fruits, carbs cannot harm your body.

Carbohydrates are only bad for your health and weight when you are consuming them in excessive amounts, without eating vegetables, fruits, and good fats.

In that case, your body will only focus on burning the carbs to create glucose (the essential brain's energy supply) whiles the fats remain stored in layers around your stomach, arms, and legs.

The more straightforward answer to the chapter's title is that there is no defined Mediterranean Diet. You can't expect people in Italy to eat the same meals as people in France or Spain, for example.

The similarity lies in the way these people fill their plates and, most importantly, what ingredients they use.

Although it is called a Mediterranean Diet, it is, in fact, an eating pattern. It is not a diet in the literal meaning of the word. For this reason, people love it and tend to accept it much better than any other diet that strictly tells you what you can and cannot eat.

It is up to you to see what foods are suitable for your body, how many calories you need to lose, what activities are necessary for you to bring your body in good shape. This is how you will create your Mediterranean diet menu.

The so-called Mediterranean diet pyramid is the best indicator that will help you start and create every meal of your day.

This pyramid puts an accent on consuming vegetables, fruits, whole grains, nuts, olive oil, herbs and spices, fish, seafood, beans, and legumes at least five times in the week. Eggs, cheese, poultry, and yogurt should be consumed in moderate amounts, while sweets, soda drinks, heavy liquor, and red meat are reserved only for special occasions.

What is impressive about this diet is the fact that nothing is forbidden; there are priority foods and foods that should be eaten less frequently.

When it comes to alcoholic drinks, this diet is allowing red wine, but only in moderation. One glass of red wine is more than enough for women, and two for men; but, wine is not a must. Include it if you feel like drinking it and if your doctor allows it.

The most important part is to include physical activity several times per week. You can start with something light, such as simple hiking or walking instead of using your car or the bus.

If typical exercising is not your favorite thing, and you don't feel like hiking or walking, you can always add something else, such as dancing classes or even gardening.

CHAPTER 1:

About the Mediterranean Diet

The Mediterranean diet is full of never-ending varieties of healthy, fresh, and delicious foods. However, there is more of an emphasis on certain types of foods, nothing is excluded. People who try a Mediterranean diet can enjoy the dishes they love while also learning to appreciate how good the freshest, healthiest foods can be. Transitioning into the Mediterranean diet is mainly about bracing yourself for a new way of eating, adapting your attitude toward food into one of joyful expectation and appreciation of good meals and good company. It's like a mindset as anything else, so you'll want to make your environment unite so you can quickly adapt to the lifestyle in the Mediterranean way.

Benefits of the Mediterranean Diet

Boosts Your Brain Health: Preserve memory and prevent cognitive decline by following the Mediterranean diet that will limit processed foods, refined bread, and red meats. Have a glass of wine versus hard liquor.

Improves Poor Eyesight: Older individuals suffer from poor eyesight, but in many cases, the Mediterranean diet has provided notable improvement. An Australian Center for Eye Research discovered that the individuals who consumed a minimum of 100 ml (0.42 cup) of olive oil weekly were almost 50% less likely to develop macular degeneration versus those who ate less than one ml each week.

Helps to Reduce the Risk of Heart Disease: The New England Journal of Medicine provided evidence in 2013 from a randomized clinical trial. The trial was implemented in Spain, whereas individuals did not have cardiovascular disease at enrollment but were in the 'high risk' category. The incidence of major cardiovascular events was reduced by the Mediterranean diet that was supplemented with extra-virgin olive oil or nuts. In one study, men who consumed fish in this manner reduced the risk by 23% of death from heart disease.

The Risk of Alzheimer's disease is reduced: In 2018, the journal Neurology studied 70 brain scans of individuals who had no signs of dementia at the onset. They followed the eating patterns in a two-year study resulting in individuals who were on the Med diet had a lesser increase of the depots and reduced energy use - potentially signaling risk for Alzheimer's.

Helps Lessen the Risk of Some Types of Cancer: According to the results of a group study, the diet is associated with a lessened risk of stomach cancer (gastric adenocarcinoma).

Decreases Risks for Type 2 Diabetes: It can help stabilize blood sugar while protecting against type 2 diabetes with its low-carb elements. The Med diet maintains a richness in fiber, which will digest slowly while preventing variances in your blood sugar. It also can help you maintain a healthier weight, which is another trigger for diabetes.

Suggests Improvement for Those with Parkinson's disease: By consuming foods on the Mediterranean diet, you add high levels of antioxidants that can prevent your body from undergoing oxidative stress, which is a damaging process that will attack your cells. The menu plan can reduce your risk factors in half.

Mediterranean Diet Pyramid

The Mediterranean Diet Pyramid is a nutritional guide developed by the World Health Organization, Harvard School of Public Health, and Oldways Preservation Trust in 1993. It is a visual tool that summarizes the Mediterranean diet, suggested eating patterns, and guides how frequently specific mechanisms should be eaten. It allows you to break healthy eating habits and not overfill yourself with too many calories.

Olive oil, fruits, vegetables, whole grains, legumes, beans, nuts & seeds, spices & herbs: These foods form the Mediterranean pyramid base. If you did observe, you would notice that these are mostly from plant sources. You should try and include a few variations of these items into each meal you eat. Olive oil should be the primary fat in cooking your dishes and endeavor to replace any other butter or cooking oil you may have been using to cook.

Fish & seafood: These are essential staples of the Mediterranean diet that should be consumed often as a protein source. You would want to include these in your diet at least two times a week. Try new varieties of fish, either frozen or fresh. Also, incorporate seafood like mussels, crab, and shrimp into your diet. Canned tuna is also great to include on sandwiches or toss in a salad with fresh vegetables.

Cheese, yogurt, eggs & poultry: These ingredients should be consumed in more moderate amounts. Depending on the food, they should be used sparingly throughout the week. Keep in mind that if you are using eggs in baking or cooking, they will also be counted in your weekly limit. You would want to stick to more healthy cheese like Parmesan, ricotta, or feta that you can add a topping or garnish on your dishes.

Red meat & sweets: These items are going to be consumed less frequently. If you are going to eat them, you need to consume only small quantities, most preferably lean meat versions with less fat when possible. Most studies recommend a maximum of 12 to 16 ounces per month. To add more variety to your diet, you can still have red meat occasionally, but you would want to reduce how often you have it. It is essential to limit its intake because of all the health concerns of sugar and red meat. The Mediterranean diet improves cardiovascular health and reduces blood pressure, while red meat tends to be dangerous to your cardiovascular system. The Greece population ate very little red meat and instead had fish or seafood as their main protein source.

Water: The Mediterranean diet encourages you to stay hydrated at all times. It means drinking more water than your daily intake. The Institute of Medicine recommends a total of 9 cups each day for women and 13 cups for men. For pregnant or breastfeeding women, the number should be increased.

Wine: Moderate consumption of wine with meals is encouraged on the Mediterranean diet. Studies shown that moderate consumption of alcohol can reduce the risk of heart disease. That can mean about 1 glass per day for women. Men tend to have higher body mass so that they can consume 1 to 2 drinks. Please keep in mind what your doctor would recommend regarding wine consumption based on your health and family history.

CHAPTER 2:

The History of the Mediterranean Diet

Just like it sounds, the Mediterranean diet comes from the dietary traditions of the people of the Mediterranean isle region such as the Romans and Greeks. The people of these regions had a rich diet full of fruits, bread, wine, olive oil, nuts, and seafood. Despite the fatty elements in their diet, the people of this region tended to live longer and overall healthy lives with relatively less cardiovascular heart issues. This phenomenon was noticed by American scientist Ancel Keys in the 1950s.

Keys was an academic researcher at the University of Minnesota in the 1950s who researched healthy eating habits and how to reverse the decline in American cardiovascular health. He found in his research that poor people in the Mediterranean region of the world were healthier compared to the rich American population which had seen a recent rise in cardiovascular heart issues and obesity. Compared to wealthy New Yorkers, the lower class in the Mediterranean lived well into their 90s and tended to be physically active in their senior years. Keys and his team of scientists decided to travel the world and study the link between the region's diet and the health of the people who lived there. In 1957, he traveled and studied the lifestyles, nutrition, exercise, and diet of the United States, Italy, Holland, Greece, Japan, Finland, and Yugoslavia.

Keys' research found that the dietary choices of the people from the Mediterranean region allowed them to live a longer lifespan and one that kept them more physically active compared to other world populations. The people of Greece, in particular, ate a diet that consisted of healthy fats like seafood, nuts, olive oil, and fatty fish. Despite the amount of fat in these sources, their cardiovascular health stayed consistent without the risk factors for a heart attack or stroke. His study became a guideline for the United States to set its own nutritional standards, and he became known as the father of nutritional science.

With Keys' work leading the way, further research and clinical trials have been conducted on the Mediterranean diet which gives evidence for its health-improving properties. Not only will you lose weight, but you could lower your LDL "bad" cholesterol, lower your blood pressure, and decrease and stabilize blood sugar levels. With a decrease in these signs of cardiovascular heart disease, you can greatly reduce your risk of suffering from heart attack, stroke, or premature death.

It's important to point out that the Mediterranean diet cannot alone bring about these changes to someone's health. It will depend on a variety of other factors in their lifestyle such as genetics, physical exercise, smoking, obesity, drug use, etc. Part of the combination of the Mediterranean diet is incorporating physical exercise into your life. That's how it goes from the Mediterranean "diet" to a Mediterranean "lifestyle" that truly mimics the people of that region. The people of Greece tend to live an active lifestyle with some sort of daily physical activity they partake in. Whether that is walking, sailing, rowing, swimming, or hiking, coupling that physical exercise that with a healthy plant-based diet is what can bring about the beneficial health results. In our current environment, physical activity could mean a session at the gym or even just a walk around the block. It doesn't have to highly intensive, but the important part is incorporating some sort of physical activity in your day, so you can truly gain the benefits of following this diet.

Before we begin listing a rudimentary list of what you can and cannot eat, it's important to highlight that the Mediterranean region consists of many countries with their own unique dietary choices. With this diversity comes many varieties of recipes that you can incorporate into your dishes as long as you are still following the healthy tenets of the Mediterranean diet. This gives a basic outline of which foods you should include on your shopping list and then you can look for recipes from there! What does the basic Mediterranean diet look like?

- Your diet should consist heavily of whole grain bread, extra virgin olive oil, fresh fruits and vegetables, herbs and spices, nuts and seeds, fish and seafood

- You should moderately eat: poultry, cheese, egg, and yogurt

- You should try to eat: red meat and organ meat rarely

- You should avoid the following: processed snacks, refined oils (canola oil or vegetable oil), refined grains (white bread), sugary drinks (juice, soda), processed meats (hot dogs, sausages, bacon), trans fats

- You should drink: water, wine

CHAPTER 3:

What To Eat: The Mediterranean Diet Food List

The Mediterranean diet is a very beneficial diet. That said, it is very hard for you to experience any of the benefits that you have just learned without following the diet to the latter. One way of doing that is by eating what the diet allows and avoiding what the diet prohibits you to eat. Let's get started

What you can eat

The foods you can eat while you are on a Mediterranean diet fall into two categories. There are those foods that you can eat regularly and there are those that you should only eat in moderation. Here is an extensive list of both categories.

Foods to eat regularly

Healthy fats like avocado oil, avocados, olives and extra virgin olive oil

Fruits like peaches, figs, melons, dates, bananas, strawberries, grapes, pears, oranges, and apples. Note that you can eat most fruits while on this diet

Vegetables like cucumbers, Brussels sprouts, artichoke, eggplant, carrots, cauliflower, onions, spinach, kale, broccoli and tomatoes. Those are just popular examples but basically all vegetables are allowed in the Mediterranean diet

Whole grains like pasta, whole wheat, whole grain bread, corn, buckwheat, barley, rye, brown rice and whole oats.

Nuts and seeds like pumpkin seeds, cashews, pistachios, walnuts, almonds and macadamia nuts

Herbs and spices; the best herbs and spices are mostly fresh and dried like mint, rosemary, cinnamon, basil and pepper.

Tubers like sweet potatoes, yams, turnips and potatoes.

Legumes like chickpeas, peanuts, pulses, lentils, peas and beans.

Fish and seafood, which are actually your primary source of protein. Good examples include shellfish like crab, mussels and oysters, shrimp, tuna, haddock and salmon.

Foods You Should Eat In Moderation

You should only eat the below foods less frequently when compared to the foods in the list above.

Red meat like bacon, ground beef and steak

Dairy products low in fat or fat free. Some of the popular examples include cheese, yogurt and low fat milk

Eggs, as they are good sources of proteins and are healthier when poached and boiled

Poultry like duck, turkey and chicken

Note that chicken are healthy when their skin is removed. This is because you reduce the cholesterol in the chicken.

Later on in the book, this list of foods that you are allowed to eat when on a Mediterranean diet will be expanded further where you will know what foods to take on a daily, weekly and monthly basis.

Food to Avoid

The below list contains a couple of foods that you need to avoid when on a Mediterranean diet completely. This is because they are unhealthy and when you eat them, you will be unable to experience the benefits of a Mediterranean diet. These foods include;

Processed meat- you should avoid processed meats like bacon, sausage and hot dogs because they are high in saturated fats, which are unhealthy.

Refined oils - stay away from unhealthy oils like cottonseed oil, vegetable oil and soybean oil.

Saturated or Trans-fats - good example of these fats include butter and margarine.

Highly processed foods – avoid all highly processed foods. By this, I mean all the foods that are packaged. This can be packaged crisp, nuts, wheat etc. Some of these foods are marked and labeled low fat but are actually quite high in sugar.

Refined grains - avoid refined grains like refined pasta, white bread, cereals, bagels etc

Added sugar- foods, which contain added sugar like sodas, chocolates, candy and ice cream should be completely avoided. If you have a sweet tooth, you can substitute products with added sugar with natural sweeteners.

Now that you know what to eat and what not to eat when on the Mediterranean diet you are now ready to learn how you can adopt the diet. The next chapter will show you how to do that.

CHAPTER 4:

Getting Started with the Mediterranean Diet and Meal Planning

The Mediterranean diet is a straightforward, easy to follow, and delicious diet, but you need a bit of preparation. Preparing for the Mediterranean diet is largely about preparing yourself for a new way of eating and adjusting your attitude toward food into one of joyful expectation and appreciation of good meals and good company.

Planning Your Mediterranean Diet

There are a few things to make your transition to the diet easier and effortless.

Ease your way into more healthful eating:

Before starting the diet, it can be helpful to spend a week or two cutting back on the least healthful foods that you are currently eating. You might start with fast food or eliminate cream-based sauces and soups. You can begin by cutting back on processed foods like frozen meals, boxed dinners, and chips. Some other things to start trimming might be sodas, coffee with a lot of sugar, and milk. You should lower butter, and cut out red meats such as lamb, beef, and pork.

Start thinking about what you'll be eating:

Just like planning for a vacation, you need to plan your diet. Go through the list of foods you need to eat on the Mediterranean diet and get recipe and meal ideas.

Gather what you'll need:

Everything in the Mediterranean diet is easily found at farmers' markets, grocery stores, and seafood shops. Find out where your local farmers' markets are and spend a leisurely morning checking out what is available. Talk to the farmers about what they harvest and when. Building relationships with those vendors can lead to getting special deals and the best selection. You can join the CSA (Community Supported Agriculture) farm nearby. CSA farms are small farms that sell subscription packages of whatever they're growing that season.

For a moderate seasonal or weekly fee, the farm will supply you with enough of that week's harvest to feed your whole family.

Freshness is important when following the Mediterranean diet. Joining a CSA is a great way to enjoy the freshness and peak flavor that is so important to the Mediterranean diet. The same is true for your local seafood market and butcher shop. Find out who's selling the freshest, most healthful meats and seafood and buy from them.

When you're ready to start, create a shopping list and get as many of your ingredients from your new sources as you can.

Plan your week:

Planning ahead is essential to success. The diet is heavily plant-based, and you need to load up on fresh fruits, vegetables, and herbs each week. By keeping your pantry stocked with whole grains like whole-wheat pasta, polenta, dried or canned beans and legumes, olive oil, and even some canned, vegetables and fish, you can be sure that you'll always have the ingredients for a healthy meal.

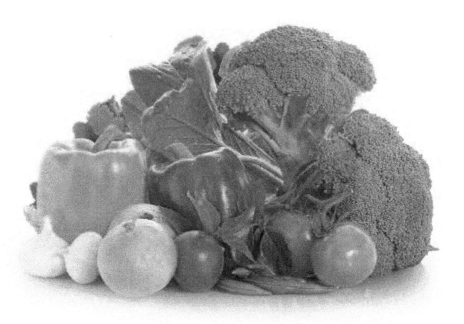

Adjust your portions:

The idea behind the Mediterranean diet is to make up the bulk of your diet with plant-based foods like fruits, vegetables, whole grains, beans, and nuts. Foods like cheese, meat, and sweets are allowed, but they are consumed only occasionally and in small portions. One way to ensure that you're eating enough plant-based foods while following the Mediterranean diet is to fill half your plate with vegetables and fruit, then fill one-quarter with whole grains, and the last quarter your plate with protein such as beans, fish, shellfish, or poultry. Once every week or two, enjoy a small serving of red meat, such as beef or lamb, or use meat as an accent to add flavor to plant-based stews, sauces, or other dishes. Here are some guidelines that will help you visualize appropriate portions for the Mediterranean diet:

- One ½ cup serving of grains or beans are about the size of the palm of your hand.
- 1 cup of vegetables is as big as a baseball.
- One medium piece of fruit is as big as a tennis ball.
- One 1-ounce serving of cheese is about the size of a pair of dice.
- One 3-ounce portion of meat (pork, lamb, fish, beef, or poultry) is roughly the size of a deck of cards.

CHAPTER 5:

Breakfast

Breakfast (Seafood Recipes)

1. Baked Bean Fish Meal

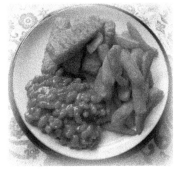

Difficulty: Novice level

Preparation Time: 10 minutes

Cooking Time: 10 minutes

Servings: 4

Size/ Portion: 1 ounce

Ingredients:

- 1 tablespoon balsamic vinegar
- 2 ½ cups green beans
- 1-pint cherry or grape tomatoes
- 4 (4-ounce each) fish fillets, such as cod or tilapia
- 2 tablespoons olive oil

Directions:

1. Preheat an oven to 400 degrees. Grease two baking sheets with some olive oil or olive oil spray. Arrange 2 fish fillets on each sheet. In a mixing bowl, pour olive oil and vinegar. Combine to mix well with each other.

2. Mix green beans and tomatoes. Combine to mix well with each other. Combine both mixtures well with each other. Add mixture equally over fish fillets. Bake for 6-8 minutes, until fish opaque and easy to flake. Serve warm.

Nutrition

229 Calories

13g Fat

2.5g Protein

1.7g Carbohydrates

2. Mushroom Cod Stew

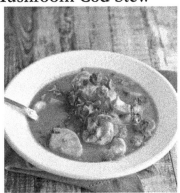

Difficulty: Novice level

Preparation Time: 10 minutes

Cooking Time: 20 minutes

Servings: 6

Size/ Portion: 2 cups

Ingredients:

- 2 tablespoons extra-virgin olive oil
- 2 garlic cloves, minced
- 1 can tomato
- 2 cups chopped onion

- ¾ teaspoon smoked paprika
- a (12-ounce) jar roasted red peppers
- 1/3 cup dry red wine
- ¼ teaspoon kosher or sea salt
- ¼ teaspoon black pepper
- 1 cup black olives
- 1 ½ pounds cod fillets, cut into 1-inch pieces
- 3 cups sliced mushrooms

Directions:

1. Get medium-large cooking pot, warm up oil over medium heat. Add onions and stir-cook for 4 minutes.
2. Add garlic and smoked paprika; cook for 1 minute, stirring often. Add tomatoes with juice, roasted peppers, olives, wine, pepper, and salt; stir gently.
3. Boil mixture. Add the cod and mushrooms; turn down heat to medium. Close and cook until the cod is easy to flake, stir in between. Serve warm.

Nutrition 238 Calories 7g Fat

3.5g Protein 8.3g Carbohydrates

3.   Spiced Swordfish

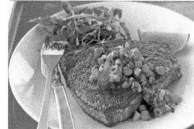

Difficulty: Novice level

Preparation Time: 10 minutes

Cooking Time: 15 minutes

Servings: 4

Size/ Portion: 7 ounces

Ingredients:

- 4 (7 ounces each) swordfish steaks

- 1/2 teaspoon ground black pepper
- 12 cloves of garlic, peeled
- 3/4 teaspoon salt
- 1 1/2 teaspoon ground cumin
- 1 teaspoon paprika
- 1 teaspoon coriander
- 3 tablespoons lemon juice
- 1/3 cup olive oil

Directions:

1. Take a blender or food processor, open the lid and add all the ingredients except for swordfish. Close the lid and blend to make a smooth mixture. Pat dry fish steaks; coat evenly with the prepared spice mixture.
2. Add them over an aluminum foil, cover and refrigerator for 1 hour. Preheat a griddle pan over high heat, pour oil and heat it. Add fish steaks; stir-cook for 5-6 minutes per side until cooked through and evenly browned. Serve warm.

Nutrition

255 Calories

12g Fat

0.5g Protein

12.7g Carbohydrates

4.   Anchovy Pasta Mania

Difficulty: Novice level

Preparation Time: 10 minutes

Cooking Time: 20 minutes

Servings: 4

Size/ Portion: 1 fillet

Ingredients:

- 4 anchovy fillets, packed in olive oil
- ½ pound broccoli, cut into 1-inch florets
- 2 cloves garlic, sliced
- 1-pound whole-wheat penne

- 2 tablespoons olive oil
- ¼ cup Parmesan cheese, grated
- Salt and black pepper, to taste
- Red pepper flakes, to taste

Directions:

1. Cook pasta as directed over pack; drain and set aside. Take a medium saucepan or skillet, add oil. Heat over medium heat.

2. Add anchovies, broccoli, and garlic, and stir-cook until veggies turn tender for 4-5 minutes. Take off heat; mix in the pasta. Serve warm with Parmesan cheese, red pepper flakes, salt, and black pepper sprinkled on top.

Nutrition

328 Calories

8g Fat

7g Protein

11.7g Carbohydrates

5.   Shrimp Garlic Pasta

Difficulty: Novice level

Preparation Time: 10 minutes

Cooking Time: 15 minutes

Servings: 4

Size/ Portion: 2 ounces

Ingredients:

- 1-pound shrimp
- 3 garlic cloves, minced
- 1 onion, finely chopped
- 1 package whole wheat or bean pasta
- 4 tablespoons olive oil
- Salt and black pepper, to taste
- ¼ cup basil, cut into strips
- ¾ cup chicken broth, low-sodium

Directions:

1. Cook pasta as directed over pack; rinse and set aside. Get medium saucepan, add oil then warm up over medium heat. Add onion, garlic and stir-cook until become translucent and fragrant for 3 minutes.

2. Add shrimp, black pepper (ground) and salt; stir-cook for 3 minutes until shrimps are opaque. Add broth and simmer for 2-3 more minutes. Add pasta in serving plates; add shrimp mixture over; serve warm with basil on top.

Nutrition

605 Calories

17g Fat

19g Protein

1.7g Carbohydrates

6.   Vinegar Honeyed Salmon

Difficulty: Novice level

Preparation Time: 10 minutes

Cooking Time: 5 minutes

Servings: 4

Size/ Portion: 8 ounces

Ingredients:

- 4 (8-ounce) salmon filets
- 1/2 cup balsamic vinegar
- 1 tablespoon honey
- Black pepper and salt, to taste
- 1 tablespoon olive oil

Directions:

1. Combine honey and vinegar. Combine to mix well with each other.

2. Season fish fillets with the black pepper (ground) and sea salt; brush with honey glaze. Take a medium saucepan or skillet, add oil.

3. Heat over medium heat. Add salmon fillets and stir-cook until medium rare in center and lightly browned for 3-4 minutes per side. Serve warm.

Nutrition

481 Calories

16g Fat

1.5g Protein

2.3gCarbohydrates

7. Orange Fish Meal

Difficulty: Novice level

Preparation Time: 10 minutes

Cooking Time: 5 minutes

Servings: 4

Size/ Portion: 4 ounces

Ingredients:

- ¼ teaspoon kosher or sea salt
- 1 tablespoon extra-virgin olive oil
- 1 tablespoon orange juice
- 4 (4-ounce) tilapia fillets, with or without skin
- ¼ cup chopped red onion
- 1 avocado, pitted, skinned, and sliced

Directions:

1. Take a baking dish of 9-inch; add olive oil, orange juice, and salt. Combine well. Add fish fillets and coat well.

2. Add onions over fish fillets. Cover with a plastic wrap. Microwave for 3 minutes until fish is cooked well and easy to flake. Serve warm with sliced avocado on top.

Nutrition

231 Calories

9g Fat

2.5g Protein

3.8g Carbohydrates

8. Shrimp Zoodles

Difficulty: Novice level

Preparation Time: 10 minutes

Cooking Time: 5 minutes

Servings: 2

Size/ Portion: 2 ounces

Ingredients:

- 2 tablespoons chopped parsley
- 2 teaspoons minced garlic
- 1 teaspoon salt
- ½ teaspoon black pepper
- 2 medium zucchinis, spiralized
- 3/4 pounds medium shrimp, peeled & deveined
- 1 tablespoon olive oil
- 1 lemon, juiced and zested

Directions:

1. Take a medium saucepan or skillet, add oil, lemon juice, lemon zest. Heat over medium heat. Add shrimps and stir-cook 1 minute per side.

2. Sauté garlic and red pepper flakes for 1 more minute. Add Zoodles and stir gently; cook for 3 minutes until cooked to satisfaction. Season well, serve warm with parsley on top.

Nutrition

329 Calories

12g Fat

3g Protein

6.5g Carbohydrates

9. Asparagus Trout Meal

Difficulty: Intermediate level

Preparation Time: 10 minutes

Cooking Time: 20 minutes

Servings: 4

Size/ Portion: ½ fillets

Ingredients:

- 2 pounds trout fillets
- 1-pound asparagus
- 1 tablespoon olive oil
- 1 garlic clove, finely minced
- 1 scallion, thinly sliced
- 4 medium golden potatoes
- 2 Roma tomatoes, chopped
- 8 pitted kalamata olives, chopped
- 1 large carrot, thinly sliced
- 2 tablespoons dried parsley
- ¼ cup ground cumin
- 2 tablespoons paprika
- 1 tablespoon vegetable bouillon seasoning
- ½ cup dry white wine

Directions:

1. In a mixing bowl, add fish fillets, white pepper and salt. Combine to mix well with each other. Take a medium saucepan or skillet, add oil.

2. Heat over medium heat. Add asparagus, potatoes, garlic, white part scallion, and stir-cook until become softened for 4-5 minutes. Add tomatoes, carrot and olives; stir-cook for 6-7 minutes until turn tender. Add cumin, paprika, parsley, bouillon seasoning, and salt. Stir mixture well.

3. Mix in white wine and fish fillets. Over low heat, cover and simmer mixture for about 6 minutes until fish is easy to flake, stir in between. Serve warm with green scallions on top.

Nutrition

303 Calories

17g Fat

6g Protein

5g Carbohydrates

10.   Kale Olive Tuna

Difficulty: Intermediate level

Preparation Time: 10 minutes

Cooking Time: 15 minutes

Servings: 6

Size/ Portion: 1 ounce

Ingredients:

- 1 cup chopped onion
- 3 garlic cloves, minced
- 1 (2.25-ounce) can sliced olives
- 1-pound kale, chopped
- 3 tablespoons extra-virgin olive oil
- ¼ cup capers
- ¼ teaspoon crushed red pepper
- 2 teaspoons sugar
- 1 (15-ounce) can cannellini beans
- 2 (6-ounce) cans tuna in olive oil, un-drained
- ¼ teaspoon black pepper
- ¼ teaspoon kosher or sea salt

Directions:

1. Soak kale in boiling water for 2 minutes; drain and set aside. Take a medium-large cooking pot or stock pot, heat oil over medium heat.

2. Add onion and stir-cook until become translucent and softened. Add garlic and stir-cook until become fragrant for 1 minute.

3. Add olives, capers, and red pepper, and stir-cook for 1 minute. Mix in cooked kale and sugar. Over low heat, cover and simmer mixture for about 8-10 minutes, stir in between.

4. Add tuna, beans, pepper, and salt. Stir well and serve warm.

Nutrition 242 Calories 11g Fat

7g Protein11.4g Carbohydrates

11. Tangy Rosemary Shrimps

Difficulty: Intermediate level

Preparation Time: 10 minutes

Cooking Time: 10 minutes

Servings: 6

Size/ Portion: ¼ ounce

Ingredients:

- 1 large orange, zested and peeled
- 3 garlic cloves, minced
- 1 ½ pounds raw shrimp, shells and tails removed
- 3 tablespoons olive oil
- 1 tablespoon chopped thyme
- 1 tablespoon chopped rosemary
- ¼ teaspoon black pepper
- ¼ teaspoon kosher or sea salt

Directions:

1. Take a zip-top plastic bag, add orange zest, shrimps, 2 tablespoons olive oil, garlic, thyme, rosemary, salt, and black pepper. Shake well and set aside to marinate for 5 minutes.

2. Take a medium saucepan or skillet, add 1 tablespoon olive oil. Heat over medium heat. Add shrimps and stir-cook for 2-3 minutes per side until totally pink and opaque.

3. Slice orange into bite-sized wedges and add in a serving plate. Add shrimps and combine well. Serve fresh.

Nutrition 187 Calories 7g Fat

0.5g Protein 2.4g Carbohydrates

12. Asparagus Salmon

Difficulty: Intermediate level

Preparation Time: 10 minutes

Cooking Time: 15 minutes

Servings: 2

Size/ Portion: 1 fillet

Ingredients:

- 8.8-ounce bunch asparagus
- 2 small salmon fillets
- 1 ½ teaspoon salt
- 1 teaspoon black pepper
- 1 tablespoon olive oil
- 1 cup hollandaise sauce, low-carb

Directions:

1. Season well the salmon fillets. Take a medium saucepan or skillet, add oil. Heat over medium heat.

2. Add salmon fillets and stir-cook until evenly seared and cooked well for 4-5 minutes per side. Add asparagus and stir cook for 4-5 more minutes. Serve warm with hollandaise sauce on top.

Nutrition

565 Calories

7g Fat

2.5g Protein

11.5g Carbohydrates

13. Tuna Nutty Salad

Difficulty: Intermediate level

Preparation Time: 10 minutes

Cooking Time: 0 minutes

Servings: 4

Size/ Portion: 2 ounces

Ingredients:

- 1 tablespoon chopped tarragon
- 1 stalk celery, trimmed and finely diced
- 1 medium shallot, diced
- 3 tablespoons chopped chives
- 1 (5-ounce) can tuna (covered in olive oil)
- 1 teaspoon Dijon mustard
- 2-3 tablespoons mayonnaise

- 1/4 teaspoon salt
- 1/8 teaspoon pepper
- 1/4 cup pine nuts, toasted

Directions:

1. In a large salad bowl, add tuna, shallot, chives, tarragon, and celery. Combine to mix well with each other. In a mixing bowl, add mayonnaise, mustard, salt, and black pepper.
2. Combine to mix well with each other. Add mayonnaise mixture to salad bowl; toss well to combine. Add pine nuts and toss again. Serve fresh.

Nutrition

236 Calories

14g Fat 1g Protein

6.3g Carbohydrates

14. Creamy Shrimp Soup

Difficulty: Professional level

Preparation Time: 10 minutes

Cooking Time: 35 minutes

Servings: 6

Size/ Portion: 2 cups

Ingredients:

- 1-pound medium shrimp
- 1 leek, both whites and light green parts, sliced
- 1 medium fennel bulb, chopped
- 2 tablespoons olive oil
- 3 stalks celery, chopped
- 1 clove garlic, minced
- Sea salt and ground pepper to taste
- 4 cups vegetable or chicken broth
- 1 tablespoon fennel seeds
- 2 tablespoons light cream
- Juice of 1 lemon

Directions:

1. Take a medium-large cooking pot or Dutch oven, heat oil over medium heat. Add celery, leek, and fennel and stir-cook for about 15 minutes, until vegetables are softened and browned. Add garlic; season with black pepper and sea salt to taste. Add fennel seed and stir.
2. Pour broth and bring to a boil. Over low heat, simmer mixture for about 20 minutes, stir in between. Add shrimp and cook until just pink for 3 minutes. Mix in cream and lemon juice; serve warm.

Nutrition

174 Calories

5g Fat

2g Protein

4.6g Carbohydrates

15. Spiced Salmon with Vegetable Quinoa

Difficulty: Professional level

Preparation Time: 30 minutes

Cooking Time: 10 minutes

Servings: 4

Size/ Portion: 5 ounces

Ingredients:

- 1 cup uncooked quinoa
- 1 teaspoon of salt, divided in half
- ¾ cup cucumbers, seeds removed, diced
- 1 cup of cherry tomatoes, halved
- ¼ cup red onion, minced
- 4 fresh basil leaves, cut in thin slices
- Zest from one lemon
- ¼ teaspoon black pepper
- 1 teaspoon cumin
- ½ teaspoon paprika
- 4 (5-g) salmon fillets

- 8 lemon wedges
- ¼ cup fresh parsley, chopped

Directions:

1. To a medium-sized saucepan, add the quinoa, 2 cups of water, and ½ teaspoons of the salt. Heat these until the water is boiling, then lower the temperature until it is simmering. Cover the pan and let it cook 20 minutes or as long as the quinoa package instructs. Turn off the burner under the quinoa and allow it to sit, covered, for at least another 5 minutes before serving.

2. Right before serving, add the onion, tomatoes, cucumbers, basil leaves, and lemon zest to the quinoa and use a spoon to stir everything together gently. In the meantime (while the quinoa cooks), prepare the salmon. Turn on the oven broiler to high and make sure a rack is in the lower part of the oven. To a small bowl, add the following components: black pepper, ½ teaspoon

of the salt, cumin, and paprika. Stir them together.

3. Place foil over the top of a glass or aluminum baking sheet, then spray it with nonstick cooking spray. Place salmon fillets on the foil. Rub the spice mixture over each fillet (about ½ teaspoons of the spice mixture per fillet). Add the lemon wedges to the pan edges near the salmon.

4. Cook the salmon under the broiler for 8-10 minutes. Your goal is for the salmon to flake apart easily with a fork. Sprinkle the salmon with the parsley, then serve it with the lemon wedges and vegetable parsley. Enjoy!

Nutrition

385 Calories

12.5g Fat

35.5g Protein

3.8g Carbohydrates

Breakfast (Vegetable Recipes)

1. Greek Stuffed Collard Greens

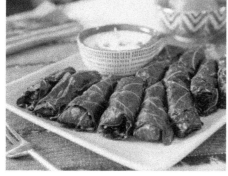

Difficulty: Novice level

Preparation Time: 10 minutes

Cooking Time: 20 minutes

Serving: 4

Size/ Portion: 5 ounces

Ingredients:

- 1 (28-ounce) can low-sodium crushed tomatoes

- 8 collard green leaves
- 2 (10-ounce) bags frozen grain medley
- 2 tablespoons grated Parmesan cheese

Direction:

1. Preheat the oven to 400°F. Pour the tomatoes into a baking pan and set aside.

2. Fill a large stockpot about three-quarters of the way with water and bring to a boil. Add the collard greens and cook for 2 minutes. Drain in a colander. Put the greens on a clean towel or paper towels and blot dry.

3. To assemble the stuffed collards, lay one leaf flat on the counter vertically. Add about ½ cup of the lentils and rice mixture to the middle of the leaf, and spread it evenly along the middle of the leaf. Fold one long side of the leaf over the rice filling, then fold over the other

long side so it is slightly overlapping. Take the bottom end, where the stem was, and gently but firmly roll up until you have a slightly square package. Carefully transfer the stuffed leaf to the baking pan, and place it seam-side down in the crushed tomatoes. Repeat with the remaining leaves.

4. Sprinkle the leaves with the grated cheese, and cover the pan with aluminum foil. Bake for 20 minutes, or until the collards are tender-firm, and serve.

Nutrition:

205 Calories 8g Fat

6g Protein 4g Carbohydrates

2. Walnut Pesto Zoodles

Difficulty: Novice level

Preparation Time: 15 minutes

Cooking Time: 10 minutes

Serving: 4

Size/ Portion: 2 cups

Ingredients:

- 4 medium zucchinis
- ¼ cup extra-virgin olive oil, divided
- 2 garlic cloves
- ½ teaspoon crushed red pepper
- ¼ teaspoon black pepper, divided
- ¼ teaspoon kosher or sea salt
- 2 tablespoons grated Parmesan cheese
- 1 cup packed fresh basil leaves
- ¾ cup walnut pieces, divided

Direction:

1. Make the zucchini noodles (zoodles) using a spiralizer or your vegetable peeler to make ribbons. Mix zoodles with 1 tablespoon of oil, 1 minced garlic clove, all the crushed red pepper, 1/8 teaspoon of black pepper, and 1/8 teaspoon of salt. Set aside.

2. In a large skillet over medium-high heat, heat ½ tablespoon of oil. Add half of the zoodles to the pan and cook for 5 minutes, stirring every minute or so. Pour the cooked zoodles into a large serving bowl, and repeat with another ½ tablespoon of oil and the remaining zoodles. Add those zoodles to the serving bowl when they are done cooking.

3. While the zoodles are cooking, make the pesto. Using a high-powered blender, add the 2 tablespoons of oil first and then the rest of the pesto ingredients. Pulse until the pesto is completely blended.

4. Add the pesto to the zoodles along with the remaining 1 tablespoon of Parmesan and the remaining ½ cup of walnuts. Mix together well and serve.

Nutrition

301 Calories 28g Fat

7g Protein 6g Carbohydrates

3. Cauliflower Steaks with Eggplant Relish

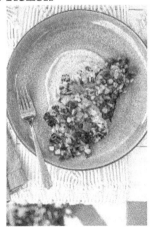

Difficulty: Novice level

Preparation Time: 5 minutes

Cooking Time: 25 minutes

Serving: 4

Size/ Portion: ½ lb.

- 2 small heads cauliflower
- ¼ teaspoon kosher or sea salt
- ¼ teaspoon smoked paprika
- extra-virgin olive oil, divided
- 1 recipe Eggplant Relish Spread

Direction:

1. Situate large, rimmed baking sheet in the oven. Set oven to 400°F with the pan inside.

2. Stand one head of cauliflower on a cutting board, stem-end down. With a long chef's knife, slice down through the very center of the head, including the stem. Starting at the cut edge, measure about 1 inch and cut one thick slice from each cauliflower half, including as much of the stem as possible, to make two cauliflower "steaks." Reserve the remaining cauliflower for another use. Repeat with the second cauliflower head.

3. Dry each steak well with a clean towel. Sprinkle the salt and smoked paprika evenly over both sides of each cauliflower steak.

4. Put skillet over medium-high heat, cook 2 tablespoons of oil. When the oil is very hot, add two cauliflower steaks to the pan and cook for about 3 minutes. Flip and cook for 2 more minutes. Transfer the steaks to a plate. Wipe out the pan to remove most of the hot oil. Repeat the cooking process with the remaining 2 tablespoons of oil and the remaining two steaks.

5. Using oven mitts, carefully remove the baking sheet from the oven and place the cauliflower on the baking sheet. Roast in the oven for 13 minutes. Serve with the Eggplant Relish Spread.

Nutrition:

282 calories 22g Fat

8g Protein

7.1g Carbohydrates

4. Mediterranean Lentil Sloppy Joes

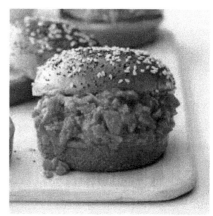

Difficulty: Novice level

Preparation Time: 5 minutes

Cooking Time: 15 minutes

Serving: 4

Size/ Portion: 2 cups

Ingredients:

- 1 tablespoon extra-virgin olive oil
- 1 cup chopped onion
- 1 cup chopped bell pepper
- 2 garlic cloves
- 1 (15-ounce) can lentils, drained and rinsed
- 1 (14.5-ounce) can low-sodium tomatoes
- 1 teaspoon ground cumin
- 1 teaspoon dried thyme
- ¼ teaspoon kosher or sea salt
- 4 whole-wheat pita breads, split open
- 1½ cups chopped seedless cucumber
- 1 cup chopped romaine lettuce

Direction

1. In a saucepan at medium-high heat, sauté onion and bell pepper for 4 minutes. Cook garlic and stir in lentils, tomatoes (with their liquid), cumin, thyme, and salt.

2. Turn the heat to medium and cook, stirring occasionally, for 10 minutes.

3. Stuff the lentil mixture inside each pita. Lay the cucumbers and lettuce on top of mixture and serve.

Nutrition:

334 Calories

5g Fat

16g Protein

2.5g Carbohydrates

5. Gorgonzola Sweet Potato Burgers

Difficulty: Novice level

Preparation Time: 10 minutes

Cooking Time: 15 minutes

Serving: 4

Size/ Portion: 1 burger

Ingredients:

- 1 large sweet potato (about 8 ounces)

- 2 tablespoons extra-virgin olive oil, divided

- 1 cup chopped onion (about ½ medium onion)

- 1 cup old-fashioned rolled oats

- 1 large egg

- 1 tablespoon balsamic vinegar

- 1 tablespoon dried oregano

- 1 garlic clove

- ¼ teaspoon kosher or sea salt

- ½ cup crumbled Gorgonzola

Direction

1. Prick sweet potato all over and microwave on high for 4 to 5 minutes. Cool slightly, then slice in half.

2. While the sweet potato is cooking, in a large skillet over medium-high heat, heat 1 tablespoon of oil. Cook onion

3. Using a spoon, carefully scoop the sweet potato flesh out of the skin and put the flesh in a food processor. Blend onion, oats, egg, vinegar, oregano, garlic, and salt. Add the cheese and pulse four times to barely combine. With your hands, form the mixture into four (½-cup-size) burgers. Place the burgers on a plate, and press to flatten each to about ¾-inch thick.

4. Clean out the skillet with a paper towel, then heat the remaining 1 tablespoon of oil over medium-high heat until very hot, about 2 minutes. Add the burgers to the hot oil, then turn the heat down to medium. Cook the burgers for 5 minutes, flip with a spatula, then cook an additional 5 minutes. Enjoy as is or serve on salad greens or whole-wheat rolls.

Nutrition:

223 Calories

13g Fat

7g Protein

8.6g Carbohydrates

6. Zucchini-Eggplant Gratin

Difficulty: Novice level

Preparation Time: 10 minutes

Cooking Time: 20 minutes

Serving: 6

Size/ Portion: 1 cup

Ingredients:

- 1 large eggplant

- 2 large zucchinis

- ¼ teaspoon black pepper

- ¼ teaspoon kosher or sea salt

- 3 tablespoons extra-virgin olive oil

- 1 tablespoon all-purpose flour

- ¾ cup 2% milk

- 1/3 cup Parmesan cheese

- 1 cup chopped tomato
- 1 cup diced or shredded fresh mozzarella
- ¼ cup fresh basil leaves

Direction:

1. Preheat the oven to 425°F.
2. Mix eggplant, zucchini, pepper, and salt.
3. Situate skillet over medium-high heat, heat 1 tablespoon of oil. Add half the veggie mixture to the skillet. Stir a few times, then cover and cook for 5 minutes, stirring occasionally. Pour the cooked veggies into a baking dish. Situate skillet back on the heat, add 1 tablespoon of oil, and repeat with the remaining veggies. Add the veggies to the baking dish.
4. While the vegetables are cooking, heat the milk in the microwave for 1 minute. Set aside.
5. Place a medium saucepan over medium heat. Add the remaining tablespoon of oil and flour, and whisk together for about 1 minute
6. Slowly pour the warm milk into the oil mixture, whisking the entire time. Add 1/3 cup of Parmesan cheese, and whisk until melted. Pour the cheese sauce over the vegetables in the baking dish and mix well.
7. Gently mix in the tomatoes and mozzarella cheese. Roast in the oven for 10 minutes, or until the gratin is almost set and not runny. Garnish with the fresh basil leaves and the remaining 2 tablespoons of Parmesan cheese before serving.

Nutrition:

207 Calories

14g Fat

11g Protein

4.8g Carbohydrates

7. Grilled Stuffed Portobello Mushrooms

Difficulty: Novice level

Preparation Time: 5 minutes

Cooking Time: 25 minutes

Serving: 6

Size/ Portion: ½ cups

Ingredients:

- 3 tablespoons extra-virgin olive oil
- 1 cup diced onion
- 2 garlic cloves
- 3 cups chopped mushrooms
- 2 small zucchinis
- 1 cup chopped tomato
- 1 teaspoon dried oregano
- ¼ teaspoon crushed red pepper
- ¼ teaspoon kosher or sea salt
- 6 large portobello mushrooms
- 4 ounces fresh mozzarella cheese
- Additional dried oregano, for serving (optional)

Direction:

1. Position skillet over medium heat, heat 2 tablespoons of oil. Add the onion and cook for 4 minutes, stirring occasionally. Stir in the garlic and cook for 1 minute, stirring often.
2. Stir in the mushrooms, zucchini, tomato, oregano, crushed red pepper, and salt. Cook for 10 minutes, stirring occasionally. Remove from the heat.
3. While the veggies are cooking, heat the grill or grill pan to medium-high heat.
4. Brush the remaining tablespoon of oil over the portobello mushroom caps. Place the mushrooms bottom-side (where the stem was removed) down on the grill or pan. Cover and cook for 5 minutes.

5. Flip the mushroom caps over, and spoon about ½ cup of the cooked vegetable mixture into each cap. Top each with about 2½ tablespoons of mozzarella and additional oregano, if desired.

6. Cover and grill for 4 to 5 minutes.

7. Remove each portobello with a spatula, and let them sit for about 5 minutes to cool slightly before serving.

Nutrition:

171 Calories

12g Fat

9g Protein

3.4g Carbohydrates

8. Stuffed Tomatoes with Tabbouleh

Difficulty: Novice level

Preparation Time: 10 minutes

Cooking Time: 20 minutes

Serving: 4

Size/ Portion: 2 pieces

Ingredients:

- 8 medium beefsteak tomatoes
- 3 tablespoons extra-virgin olive oil
- ½ cup water
- ½ cup whole-wheat couscous
- 1½ cups minced fresh curly parsley
- 1/3 cup minced fresh mint
- 2 scallions
- ¼ teaspoon black pepper
- ¼ teaspoon kosher or sea salt
- 1 medium lemon
- 4 teaspoons honey
- 1/3 cup chopped almonds

Direction:

1. Preheat the oven to 400°F.

2. Cut top off each tomato and set aside. Spoon out all the flesh inside, and put the tops, flesh, and seeds in a large mixing bowl.

3. Grease a baking dish with 1 tablespoon of oil. Place the carved-out tomatoes in the baking dish, and cover with aluminum foil. Roast for 10 minutes.

4. While the tomatoes are cooking, make the couscous by bringing the water to boil in a medium saucepan. Pour in the couscous, remove from the heat, and cover. Let sit for 5 minutes, then stir with a fork.

5. While the couscous is cooking, chop up the tomato flesh and tops. Drain off the excess tomato water using a colander. Measure out 1 cup of the chopped tomatoes (reserve any remaining chopped tomatoes for another use). Add the cup of tomatoes back into the mixing bowl. Mix in the parsley, mint, scallions, pepper, and salt.

6. Using a Micro plane or citrus grater, zest the lemon into the mixing bowl. Halve the lemon, and squeeze the juice through a strainer (to catch the seeds) from both halves into the bowl with the tomato mixture. Mix well.

7. When the couscous is ready, add it to the tomato mixture and mix well.

8. With oven mitts, carefully remove the tomatoes from the oven. Divide the tabbouleh evenly among the tomatoes and stuff them, using a spoon to press the filling down so it all fits. Wrap with the foil and return it to the oven. Cook for another 8 to 10 minutes. Before serving, top each tomato with a drizzle of ½ teaspoon of honey and about 2 teaspoons of almonds.

Nutrition:

314 Calories 15g Fat

8g Protein

2.1g Carbohydrates

9. Polenta with Mushroom Bolognese

Difficulty: Intermediate level

Preparation Time: 5 minutes

Cooking Time: 25 minutes

Serving: 4

Size/ Portion: 2 ounces

Ingredients:

- 2 (8-ounce) packages white button mushrooms
- 3 tablespoons extra-virgin olive oil, divided
- 1½ cups onion
- ½ cup carrot
- 4 garlic cloves
- 1 (18-ounce) tube plain polenta
- ¼ cup tomato paste
- 1 tablespoon dried oregano
- ¼ teaspoon ground nutmeg
- ¼ teaspoon kosher or sea salt
- ¼ teaspoon freshly ground black pepper
- ½ cup dry red wine
- ½ cup whole milk
- ½ teaspoon sugar

Direction:

1. Situate half the mushrooms in a food processor bowl and pulse about 15 times. Do with the remaining mushrooms and set aside.

2. Situate stockpot over medium-high heat, heat 2 tablespoons of oil. Cook onion and carrot then mushrooms and garlic for 10 minutes.

3. While cooking, add the remaining 1 tablespoon of oil to skillet at medium-high heat. Put 4 slices of polenta to the skillet and cook for 3 to 4 minutes. Remove the polenta from the skillet, place it on a shallow serving dish, and cover with aluminum foil to keep warm. Repeat with the remaining 4 slices of polenta.

4. To the mushroom mixture in the stockpot, add the tomato paste, oregano, nutmeg, salt, and pepper and stir. Continue cooking for another 2 to 3 minutes. Add the wine and cook for 1 to 2 minutes. Lower the heat to medium.

5. Meanwhile, in a small, microwave-safe bowl, mix the milk and sugar together and microwave on high for 30 to 45 seconds. Simmer the milk into the mushroom mixture. Drizzle the mushroom veggie sauce over the warm polenta slices.

Nutrition:

300 Calories

12g Fat

9g Protein

8.7g Carbohydrates

10. North African Peanut Stew over Cauliflower Rice

Difficulty: Intermediate level

Preparation Time: 5 minutes

Cooking Time: 25 minutes

Serving: 4

Size/ Portion: 2 cups

Ingredients:

- 1 cup frozen corn
- 2 tablespoons extra-virgin olive oil
- 1 cup chopped onion
- 2 medium Yukon Gold potatoes
- 1 large sweet potato
- 3 garlic cloves
- 1½ teaspoons ground cumin
- 1 teaspoon ground allspice
- 1 teaspoon freshly grated ginger root

- ½ teaspoon crushed red pepper
- ¼ teaspoon kosher or sea salt
- ½ cup water
- 1 (28-ounce) can diced tomatoes, undrained
- 1 (12-ounce) package frozen plain cauliflower rice
- 1 (15-ounce) can lentils, undrained
- 1/3 cup creamy peanut butter

Direction:

1. Put the corn on the counter to partially thaw while making the stew.

2. In a large stockpot over medium-high heat, heat the oil. Add the onion, potatoes, and sweet potatoes. Cook for 7 minutes. Move the potatoes to the edges of the pot, and add the garlic, cumin, allspice, ginger, crushed red pepper, and salt. Cook for 1 minute, stirring constantly. Stir in the water and cook for 1 more minute, scraping up the crispy bits from the bottom of the pan.

3. Add the tomatoes with their juices to the stockpot. Cook for 15 minutes uncovered, stirring occasionally.

4. While the tomatoes are cooking, cook the cauliflower rice according to the package directions.

5. Into the tomato mixture, stir in the lentils, partially thawed corn, and peanut butter. Adjust to medium heat and cook for 1 to 2 minutes. Serve over the cauliflower rice with hot peppers, peanuts, and fresh cilantro, if desired.

Nutrition:

467 Calories

20g Fat

21g Protein

3.8g Carbohydrates

11.   Italian Baked Beans

Difficulty: Intermediate level

Preparation Time: 5 minutes

Cooking Time: 15 minutes

Serving: 6

Size/ Portion: 2 cups

Ingredients:

- 2 teaspoons extra-virgin olive oil
- ½ cup minced onion
- 1 (12-ounce) can low-sodium tomato paste
- ¼ cup red wine vinegar
- 2 tablespoons honey
- ¼ teaspoon ground cinnamon
- ½ cup water
- 2 (15-ounce) cans cannellini

Direction:

1. Position saucepan over medium heat, heat the oil. Cook onion. Add the tomato paste, vinegar, honey, cinnamon, and water, and mix well. Turn the heat to low.

2. Drain and rinse one can of the beans in a colander and add to the saucepan. Pour the entire second can of beans (including the liquid) into the saucepan. Let it cook for 10 minutes, stirring occasionally, and serve.

Nutrition:

236 Calories

3g Fat

10g Protein

11g Carbohydrates

12.   Cannellini Bean Lettuce Wraps

Difficulty: Intermediate level

Preparation Time: 10 minutes

Cooking Time: 10 minutes

Serving: 4

Size/ portion: 2 wraps

Ingredients:

- 1 tablespoon extra-virgin olive oil
- ½ cup diced red onion
- ¾ cup chopped fresh tomatoes
- ¼ teaspoon freshly ground black pepper
- 1 (15-ounce) can cannellini beans
- ¼ cup curly parsley
- ½ cup Lemony Garlic Hummus
- 8 romaine lettuce leaves

Direction:

1. Position skillet over medium heat, heat the oil. Add the onion and cook for 3 minutes, stirring occasionally. Add the tomatoes and pepper and cook for 3 more minutes, stirring occasionally. Add the beans and cook for 3 more minutes, stirring occasionally. Pullout from the heat, and mix in the parsley.

2. Spread 1 tablespoon of hummus over each lettuce leaf. Evenly spread the warm bean mixture down the center of each leaf. Fold one side of the lettuce leaf over the filling lengthwise, then fold over the other side to make a wrap and serve.

Nutrition:

211 Calories 8g Fat

10g Protein 8g Carbohydrates

Breakfast (Poultry and Meat Recipes)

1.   Chicken Bruschetta Burgers

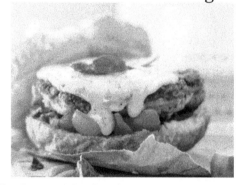

Difficulty: Novice level

Preparation Time: 10 minutes

Cooking Time: 16 minutes

Servings: 2

Ingredients:

- 1 tablespoon olive oil
- 2 garlic cloves, minced
- 3 tablespoons finely minced onion
- 1 teaspoon dried basil
- 3 tablespoons minced sun-dried tomatoes packed in olive oil
- 8 ounces (227 g) ground chicken breast
- ¼ teaspoon salt
- 3 pieces small Mozzarella balls, minced

Directions:

1. Heat the olive oil in a nonstick skillet over medium-high heat. Add the garlic and onion and sauté for 5 minutes until tender. Stir in the basil.

2. Remove from the skillet to a medium bowl.

3. Add the tomatoes, ground chicken, and salt and stir until incorporated. Mix in the Mozzarella balls.

4. Divide the chicken mixture in half and form into two burgers, each about ¾-inch thick.

5. Heat the same skillet over medium-high heat and add the burgers. Cook each side for about 5 to 6 mins. or until they reach an internal temperature of 165°F (74°C).

6. Serve warm.

Nutrition:

Calories: 300 Fat: 17.0g Protein: 32.2g

Carbs: 6.0g Fiber: 1.1g Sodium: 724mg

2. Chicken Cacciatore

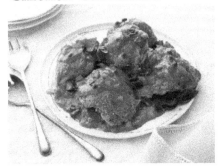

Difficulty: Novice level

Preparation Time: 15 minutes

Cooking Time: 1 hour and 30 minutes

Servings: 2

Ingredients:

- 1½ pounds (680 g) bone-in chicken thighs, skin removed and patted dry
- Salt, to taste
- 2 tablespoons olive oil
- ½ large onion, thinly sliced
- 4 ounces (113 g) baby bella mushrooms, sliced
- 1 red sweet pepper, and then cut into 1-inch pieces
- 1 (15-ounce / 425-g) can crushed fire-roasted tomatoes
- 1 fresh rosemary sprig
- ½ cup dry red wine
- 1 teaspoon Italian herb seasoning
- ½ teaspoon garlic powder
- 3 tablespoons flour

Directions:

1. Season the chicken thighs with a generous pinch of salt.
2. Heat the olive oil in a Dutch oven over medium-high heat. Add the chicken & brown for 5 minutes per side. Add the onion, mushrooms, and sweet pepper to the Dutch oven and sauté for another 5 minutes. Add the tomatoes, rosemary, wine, Italian seasoning, garlic powder, and salt, stirring well. Bring the mixture to a boil, then low the heat to low. Allow to simmer slowly for at least 1 hour, stirring occasionally, or until the chicken is tender and easily pulls away from the bone.
3. Measure out 1 cup of the sauce from the pot and put it into a bowl. Add the flour & whisk well to make a slurry.
4. Now, increase the heat to medium-high and slowly whisk the slurry into the pot. Stir until it comes to a boil and cook until the sauce is thickened.
5. Remove the chicken from the bones and shred it, and add it back to the sauce before serving, if desired.

Nutrition:

Calories: 520 Fat: 23.1g Protein: 31.8g

Carbs: 37.0g Fiber: 6.0g Sodium: 484mg

3. Chicken Gyros with Tzatziki Sauce

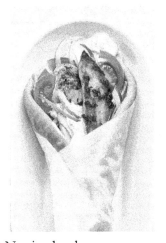

Difficulty: Novice level

Preparation Time: 15 minutes

Cooking Time: 10 minutes

Servings: 2

Ingredients:

- 2 tablespoons freshly squeezed lemon juice

- 2 tbsps. olive oil, divided, plus more for oiling the grill
- 1 teaspoon minced fresh oregano
- ½ teaspoon garlic powder
- Salt, to taste
- 8 ounces (227 g) chicken tenders
- 1 small eggplant, cut into 1-inch strips lengthwise
- 1 small zucchini, cut into ½-inch strips lengthwise
- ½ red pepper, seeded and cut in half lengthwise
- ½ English cucumber, peeled and minced
- ¾ cup plain Greek yogurt
- 1 tablespoon minced fresh dill
- 2 (8-inch) pita breads

Directions:

1. Combine the lemon juice, 1 tablespoon of olive oil, oregano, garlic powder, and salt in a medium bowl. Add the chicken and let marinate for 30 minutes.
2. Place the eggplant, zucchini, and red pepper in a large mixing bowl and sprinkle with salt and the remaining 1 tablespoon of olive oil. Toss well to coat. Let the vegetables rest while the chicken is marinating.
3. Make the tzatziki sauce: Combine the cucumber, yogurt, salt, and dill in a medium bowl. Stir well to incorporate and set aside in the refrigerator.
4. When ready, preheat the grill to medium-high heat and oil the grill grates.
5. Drain any liquid from the vegetables and put them on the grill.
6. Remove the chicken tenders from the marinade and put them on the grill.
7. Grill the chicken and vegetables for 3 minutes per side, or until the chicken is no longer pink inside.
8. Remove the chicken and vegetables from the grill and set aside. On the grill, heat the pitas for about 30 seconds, flipping them frequently.
9. Divide the chicken tenders and vegetables between the pitas and top each with ¼ cup of the prepared sauce. Roll the pitas up like a cone and serve.

Nutrition:

Calories: 586

Fat: 21.9g

Protein: 39.0g

Carbs: 62.0g

Fiber: 11.8g

Sodium: 955mg

4. Crispy Pesto Chicken

Difficulty: Novice level

Preparation Time: 15 minutes

Cooking Time: 50 minutes

Servings: 2

Ingredients:

- 12 ounces (340 g) small red potatoes (3 or 4 potatoes), scrubbed and diced into 1-inch pieces
- 1 tablespoon olive oil
- ½ teaspoon garlic powder
- ¼ teaspoon salt
- 1 (8-ounce / 227-g) boneless, skinless chicken breast
- 3 tablespoons prepared pesto

Directions:

1. Heat your oven to 425°F (220°C). Line a baking sheet with parchment paper.
2. Combine the potatoes, olive oil, garlic powder, and salt in a medium bowl. Toss well to coat.
3. Arrange the potatoes on the parchment paper and roast for 10 minutes. Flip the potatoes and roast for an additional 10 minutes.
4. Meanwhile, put the chicken in the same bowl and toss with the pesto, coating the chicken evenly.
5. Check the potatoes to make sure they are golden brown on the top and bottom. Toss them again and add the chicken breast to the pan.

6. Turn the heat down to 350°F (180°C) and roast the chicken and potatoes for 30 minutes. Check to make sure the chicken reaches an internal temperature of 165°F (74°C) and the potatoes are fork-tender.
7. Let cool for 5 minutes before serving.

Nutrition:

Calories: 378

Fat: 16.0g

Protein: 29.8g

Carbs: 30.1g

Fiber: 4.0g

Sodium: 425mg

5. Beef Stew with Beans and Zucchini

Difficulty: Novice level

Preparation Time: 20 minutes

Cooking Time: 6 to 8 hours

Servings: 2

Ingredients:

- 1 (15-ounce / 425-g) can diced or crushed tomatoes with basil
- 1 teaspoon beef base
- 2 tablespoons olive oil, divided
- 8 ounces (227 g) baby bella (cremini) mushrooms, quartered
- 2 garlic cloves, minced
- ½ large onion, diced
- 1 pound (454 g) cubed beef stew meat
- 3 tablespoons flour
- ¼ teaspoon salt
- Pinch freshly ground black pepper
- ¾ cup dry red wine
- ¼ cup minced brined olives
- 1 fresh rosemary sprig
- 1 (15-ounce / 425-g) can white cannellini beans, drained and rinsed
- One medium zucchini, cut in half lengthwise and then cut into 1-inch pieces.

Directions:

1. Place the tomatoes into a slow cooker and set it to low heat. Add the beef base and stir to incorporate.
2. Heat 1 tablespoon of olive oil in a large sauté pan over medium heat.
3. Add the mushrooms and onion and sauté for 10 minutes, stirring occasionally, or until they're golden.
4. Add the garlic and cook for 30 seconds more. Transfer the vegetables to the slow cooker.
5. In a plastic food storage bag, combine the stew meat with the flour, salt, and pepper. Seal the bag & shake well to combine.
6. Heat the remaining 1 tablespoon of olive oil in the sauté pan over high heat.
7. Add the floured meat and sear to get a crust on the outside edges. Deglaze the pan by adding about half of the red wine and scraping up any browned bits on the bottom. Stir so the wine thickens a bit and transfer to the slow cooker along with any remaining wine.
8. Stir the stew to incorporate the ingredients. Stir in the olives and rosemary, cover, and cook for 6 to 8 hours on Low.
9. About 30 minutes before the stew is finished, add the beans and zucchini to let them warm through. Serve warm.

Nutrition:

Calories: 389

Fat: 15.1g

Protein: 30.8g

Carbs: 25.0g

Fiber: 8.0g

Sodium: 582mg

6.   Greek Beef Kebabs

Difficulty: Novice level

Preparation Time: 15 minutes

Cooking Time: 20 minutes

Servings: 2

Ingredients:

- 6 ounces (170 g) beef sirloin tip, trimmed of Fat and cut into 2-inch pieces
- 3 cups of any mixture of vegetables: mushrooms, summer squash, zucchini, onions, red peppers, cherry tomatoes
- ½ cup olive oil
- ¼ cup freshly squeezed lemon juice
- 2 tablespoons balsamic vinegar
- 2 teaspoons dried oregano
- 1 teaspoon garlic powder
- 1 teaspoon salt
- 1 teaspoon minced fresh rosemary
- Cooking spray

Directions:

1. Put the beef in a plastic freezer bag.
2. Slice the vegetables into similar-size pieces and put them in a second freezer bag.
3. Make the marinade: Mix the olive oil, lemon juice, balsamic vinegar, oregano, garlic powder, salt, and rosemary in a measuring cup. Whisk well to combine. Pour half of marinade over the beef, and the other half over the vegetables.
4. Put the beef and vegetables in the refrigerator to marinate for 4 hours.
5. When ready, preheat the grill to medium-high heat and spray the grill grates with cooking spray.
6. Thread the meat onto skewers and the vegetables onto separate skewers.
7. Grill the meat for 3 mins per side. They should only take 10 to 12 minutes to cook, depending on the thickness of the meat.
8. Grill the vegetables for about 3 minutes per side, or until they have grill marks and are softened.

9. Serve hot.

Nutrition:

Calories: 284 Fat: 18.2g

Protein: 21.0g Carbs: 9.0g

Fiber: 3.9g Sodium: 122mg

7.   Chermoula   Roasted   Pork Tenderloin

Difficulty: Novice level

Preparation Time: 15 minutes

Cooking Time: 20 minutes

Servings: 2

Ingredients:

- ½ cup fresh cilantro
- ½ cup fresh parsley
- 6 small garlic cloves
- 3 tablespoons olive oil, divided
- 3 tablespoons freshly squeezed lemon juice
- 2 teaspoons cumin
- 1 teaspoon smoked paprika
- ½ teaspoon salt, divided
- Pinch freshly ground black pepper
- 1 (8-ounce / 227-g) pork tenderloin

Directions:

1. Heat your oven to 425°F (220°C).
2. In a food processor, combine the cilantro, parsley, garlic, 2 tablespoons of olive oil, lemon juice, cumin, paprika, and ¼ teaspoon of salt. Pulse 15 to 20 times, or until the mixture is fairly smooth. Scrape the sides down as needed to incorporate all the ingredients. Transfer the sauce into a small bowl & set aside.
3. Season the pork tenderloin on all sides with the remaining ¼ teaspoon of salt and a generous pinch of black pepper.
4. Heat the remaining 1 tablespoon of olive oil in a sauté pan.
5. Sear the pork for 3 minutes, turning often, until golden brown on all sides.

6. Transfer the pork into a baking dish & roast in the preheated oven for 15 minutes, or until the internal temperature registers 145°F (63°C).
7. Cool for 5 minutes before serving.

Nutrition:

Calories: 169 Fat: 13.1g

Protein: 11.0g Carbs: 2.9g

Fiber: 1.0g Sodium: 332mg

8.   Lamb Kofta (Spiced Meatballs)

Difficulty: Novice level

Preparation Time: 15 minutes

Cooking Time: 30 minutes

Servings: 2

Ingredients:

- ¼ cup walnuts
- 1 garlic clove
- ½ small onion
- 1 roasted piquillo pepper
- 2 tablespoons fresh mint
- 2 tablespoons fresh parsley
- ¼ teaspoon cumin
- ¼ teaspoon allspice
- ¼ teaspoon salt
- Pinch cayenne pepper
- 8 ounces (227 g) lean ground lamb

Directions:

1. Heat your oven to 350°F (180°C). Line a baking sheet with aluminum foil.
2. In a food processor, combine the walnuts, garlic, onion, roasted pepper, mint, parsley, cumin, allspice, salt, and cayenne pepper. Pulse about 10 times to combine everything.
3. Transfer the spice mixture to a large bowl and add the ground lamb. With your hands or a spatula, mix the spices into the lamb.
4. Roll the lamb into 1½-inch balls (about the size of golf balls).
5. Arrange the meatballs on the prepared baking sheet and bake for 30 minutes, or until cooked to an internal temperature of 165°F (74°C).
6. Serve warm.

Nutrition:

Calories: 409 Fat: 22.9g

Protein: 22.0g Carbs: 7.1g

Fiber: 3.0g Sodium: 428mg

Breakfast (Salad Recipes)

1.   Watermelon Salad

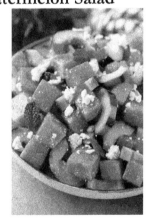

Difficulty: Novice level

Preparation Time: 18 minutes

Cooking Time: 0 minute

Serving: 6

Size/ Portion: 2 cups

Ingredients:

- ¼ teaspoon sea salt
- ¼ teaspoon black pepper
- 1 tablespoon balsamic vinegar
- 1 cantaloupe, quartered & seeded
- 12 watermelon, small & seedless
- 2 cups mozzarella balls, fresh
- 1/3 cup basil, fresh & torn
- 2 tablespoons olive oil

Directions:

1. Scoop out balls of cantaloupe, and the put them in a colander over bowl.

2. With a melon baller slice the watermelon.

3. Allow your fruit to drain for ten minutes, and then refrigerate the juice.

4. Wipe the bowl dry, and then place your fruit in it.

5. Stir in basil, oil, vinegar, mozzarella and tomatoes before seasoning.

6. Mix well and serve.

Nutrition: 218 Calories 10g Protein

13g Fat 12g Carbohydrates

2.   Orange Celery Salad

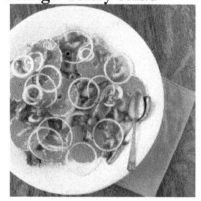

Difficulty: Novice level

Preparation Time: 16 minutes

Cooking Time: 0 minute

Serving: 6

Size/ Portion: 2 cups

Ingredients:

- 1 tablespoon lemon juice, fresh
- ¼ teaspoon sea salt, fine
- ¼ teaspoon black pepper
- 1 tablespoon olive brine
- 1 tablespoon olive oil
- ¼ cup red onion, sliced
- ½ cup green olives
- 2 oranges, peeled & sliced

- 3 celery stalks, sliced diagonally in ½ inch slices

Directions:

1. Put your oranges, olives, onion and celery in a shallow bowl.

2. Stir oil, olive brine and lemon juice, pour this over your salad.

3. Season with salt and pepper before serving.

Nutrition:

65 Calories 2g Protein

0.2g Fat 3g Carbohydrates

3.   Roasted Broccoli Salad

Difficulty: Novice level

Preparation Time: 9 minutes

Cooking Time: 17 minutes

Serving: 4

Size/ portion: 2 cups

Ingredients:

- 1 lb. broccoli
- 3 tablespoons olive oil, divided
- 1-pint cherry tomatoes
- 1 ½ teaspoons honey
- 3 cups cubed bread, whole grain
- 1 tablespoon balsamic vinegar
- ½ teaspoon black pepper
- ¼ teaspoon sea salt, fine
- grated parmesan for serving

Directions:

1. Set oven to 450, and then place rimmed baking sheet.

2. Drizzle your broccoli with a tablespoon of oil, and toss to coat.

3. Take out from oven, and spoon the broccoli. Leave oil at bottom of the bowl and add in your tomatoes, toss to coat,

then mix tomatoes with a tablespoon of honey. Place on the same baking sheet.

4. Roast for fifteen minutes, and stir halfway through your cooking time.

5. Add in your bread, and then roast for three more minutes.

6. Whisk two tablespoons of oil, vinegar, and remaining honey. Season. Pour this over your broccoli mix to serve.

Nutrition:

226 Calories 7g Protein

12g Fat 8g Carbohydrates

4.   Tomato Salad

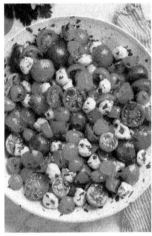

Difficulty: Novice level

Preparation Time: 22 minutes

Cooking Time: 0 minute

Serving: 4

Size/ portion: 2 cups

Ingredients:

- 1 cucumber, sliced
- ¼ cup sun dried tomatoes, chopped
- 1 lb. tomatoes, cubed
- ½ cup black olives
- 1 red onion, sliced
- 1 tablespoon balsamic vinegar
- ¼ cup parsley, fresh & chopped

- 2 tablespoons olive oil

Directions:

1. Get out a bowl and combine all of your vegetables together. To make your dressing mix all your seasoning, olive oil and vinegar.

2. Toss with your salad and serve fresh.

Nutrition

126 Calories

2.1g Protein

9.2g Fat

5.6g Carbohydrates

5.   Feta Beet Salad

Difficulty: Novice level

Preparation Time: 16 minutes

Cooking Time: 0 minute

Serving: 4

Size/ Portion: 2 cups

Ingredients:

- 6 Red Beets, Cooked & Peeled
- 3 Ounces Feta Cheese, Cubed
- 2 Tablespoons Olive Oil
- 2 Tablespoons Balsamic Vinegar

Directions:

1. Combine everything together, and then serve.

Nutrition:

230 Calories 7.3g Protein

12g Fat 11g Carbohydrates

6.   Cauliflower & Tomato Salad

Difficulty: Novice level

Preparation Time: 17 minutes

Cooking Time: 0 minute

Serving: 4

Size/ Portion: 2 cups

Ingredients:

- 1 Head Cauliflower, Chopped
- 2 Tablespoons Parsley, Fresh & chopped
- 2 Cups Cherry Tomatoes, Halved
- 2 Tablespoons Lemon Juice, Fresh
- 2 Tablespoons Pine Nuts

Directions:

1. Incorporate lemon juice, cherry tomatoes, cauliflower and parsley and season well. Sprinkle the pine nuts, and mix.

Nutrition:

64 Calories 2.8g Protein

3.3g Fat 4.5g Carbohydrates

7.   Tahini Spinach

Difficulty: Novice level

Preparation Time: 11 minutes

Cooking Time: 6 minutes

Serving: 3

Size/ Portion: 2 cups

Ingredients:

- 10 spinach, chopped
- ½ cup water
- 1 tablespoon tahini
- 2 cloves garlic, minced
- ¼ teaspoon cumin
- ¼ teaspoon paprika
- ¼ teaspoon cayenne pepper
- 1/3 cup red wine vinegar

Direction:

1. Add your spinach and water to the saucepan, and then boil it on high heat. Once boiling reduce to low, and cover. Allow it to cook on simmer for five minutes.

2. Add in your garlic, cumin, cayenne, red wine vinegar, paprika and tahini. Whisk well, and season with salt and pepper.

3. Drain your spinach and top with tahini sauce to serve.

Nutrition:

69 Calories 5g Protein

3g Fat 3.7g Carbohydrates

8.   Pilaf with Cream Cheese

Difficulty: Intermediate level

Preparation Time: 11 minutes

Cooking Time: 34 minutes

Serving: 6

Size/ Portion: 2 cups

Ingredients:

- 2 cups yellow long grain rice, parboiled
- 1 cup onion
- 4 green onions
- 3 tablespoons butter
- 3 tablespoons vegetable broth
- 2 teaspoons cayenne pepper
- 1 teaspoon paprika
- ½ teaspoon cloves, minced
- 2 tablespoons mint leaves
- 1 bunch fresh mint leaves to garnish
- 1 tablespoons olive oil

Cheese Cream:

- 3 tablespoons olive oil
- sea salt & black pepper to taste
- 9 ounces cream cheese

Directions:

1. Start by heating your oven to 360, and then get out a pan. Heat your butter and olive oil together, and cook your onions and spring onions for two minutes.

2. Add in your salt, pepper, paprika, cloves, vegetable broth, rice and remaining seasoning. S

3. Sauté for three minutes.

4. Wrap with foil, and bake for another half hour. Allow it to cool.

5. Mix in the cream cheese, cheese, olive oil, salt and pepper. Serve your pilaf garnished with fresh mint leaves.

Nutrition:

364 Calories

5g Protein

30g Fat

12g Carbohydrates

9.   Easy Spaghetti Squash

Difficulty: Intermediate level

Preparation Time: 13 minutes

Cooking Time: 45 minutes

Serving: 6

Size/ Portion: 2 ounces

Ingredients:

- 2 spring onions, chopped fine
- 3 cloves garlic, minced
- 1 zucchini, diced
- 1 red bell pepper, diced
- 1 tablespoon Italian seasoning
- 1 tomato, small & chopped fine
- 1 tablespoons parsley, fresh & chopped
- pinch lemon pepper
- dash sea salt, fine
- 4 ounces feta cheese, crumbled
- 3 Italian sausage links, casing removed
- 2 tablespoons olive oil
- 1 spaghetti sauce, halved lengthwise

Directions:

1. Prep oven to 350, and get out a large baking sheet. Coat it with cooking spray, and then put your squash on it with the cut side down.

2. Bake at 350 for forty-five minutes. It should be tender.

3. Turn the squash over, and bake for five more minutes. Scrape the strands into a larger bowl.

4. Cook tablespoon of olive oil in a skillet, and then add in your Italian sausage. Cook at eight minutes before removing it and placing it in a bowl.

5. Add another tablespoon of olive oil to the skillet and cook your garlic and onions until softened. This will take five minutes. Throw in your Italian seasoning, red peppers and zucchini. Cook for another five minutes. Your vegetables should be softened.

6. Mix in your feta cheese and squash, cooking until the cheese has melted.

7. Stir in your sausage, and then season with lemon pepper and salt. Serve with parsley and tomato.

Nutrition:

423 Calories 18g Protein

30g Fat

15g Carbohydrates

10.   Roasted Eggplant Salad

Difficulty: Intermediate level

Preparation Time: 14 minutes

Cooking Time: 36 minutes

Serving: 6

Size/ Portion: 2 cups

Ingredients:

- 1 red onion, sliced
- 2 tablespoons parsley
- 1 teaspoon thyme
- 2 cups cherry tomatoes
- 1 teaspoon oregano
- 3 tablespoons olive oil
- 1 teaspoon basil

- 3 eggplants, peeled & cubed

Directions:

1. Start by heating your oven to 350.

2. Season your eggplant with basil, salt, pepper, oregano, thyme and olive oil.

3. Arrange it on a baking tray, and bake for a half hour.

4. Toss with your remaining ingredients before serving.

Nutrition:

148 Calories

3.5g Protein

7.7g Fat

13g Carbohydrates

11.　Penne with Tahini Sauce

Difficulty: Intermediate level

Preparation Time: 16 minutes

Cooking Time: 22 minutes

Serving: 8

Size/ Portion: 2 ounces

Ingredients:

- 1/3 cup water

- 1 cup yogurt, plain

- 1/8 cup lemon juice

- 3 tablespoons tahini

- 3 cloves garlic

- 1 onion, chopped

- ¼ cup olive oil

- 2 portobello mushrooms, large & sliced

- ½ red bell pepper, diced

- 16 ounces penne pasta

- ½ cup parsley, fresh & chopped

Directions:

1. Start by getting out a pot and bring a pot of salted water to a boil. Cook your pasta al dente per package instructions.

2. Mix your lemon juice and tahini together, and then place it in a food processor. Process with garlic, water and yogurt.

3. Situate pan over medium heat. Heat up your oil, and cook your onions until soft.

4. Add in your mushroom and continue to cook until softened.

5. Add in your bell pepper, and cook until crispy.

6. Drain your pasta, and then toss with your tahini sauce, top with parsley and pepper and serve with vegetables.

Nutrition:

332 Calories

11g Proteins

12g Fat

18g Carbohydrates

12.　Roasted Veggies

Difficulty: Intermediate level

Preparation Time: 14 minutes

Cooking Time: 26 minutes

Serving: 12

Size/ Portion: 2 cups

Ingredients:

- 6 cloves garlic

- 6 tablespoons olive oil

- 1 fennel bulb, diced

- 1 zucchini, diced

- 2 red bell peppers, diced

- 6 potatoes, large & diced

- 2 teaspoons sea salt

- ½ cup balsamic vinegar

- ¼ cup rosemary, chopped & fresh

- 2 teaspoons vegetable bouillon powder

Directions:

1. Start by heating your oven to 400.

2. Get out a baking dish and place your potatoes, fennel, zucchini, garlic and fennel on a baking dish, drizzling with olive oil. Sprinkle with salt, bouillon powder, and rosemary. Mix well, and then bake at 450 for thirty to forty minutes. Mix your vinegar into the vegetables before serving.

Nutrition

675 Calories

13g Protein

21g Fat

10g Carbohydrates

13. Zucchini Pasta

Difficulty: Intermediate level

Preparation Time: 9 minutes

Cooking Time: 32 minutes

Serving: 4

Size/ Portion: 2 ounces

Ingredients:

- 3 tablespoons olive oil
- 2 cloves garlic, minced
- 3 zucchinis, large & diced
- sea salt & black pepper to taste
- ½ cup milk, 2%
- ¼ teaspoon nutmeg
- 1 tablespoon lemon juice, fresh
- ½ cup parmesan, grated
- 8 ounces uncooked farfalle pasta

Directions:

1. Get out a skillet and place it over medium heat, and then heat up the oil. Add in your garlic and cook for a minute. Stir often so that it doesn't burn. Add in your salt, pepper and zucchini. Stir well, and cook covered for fifteen minutes.

During this time, you'll want to stir the mixture twice.

2. Get out a microwave safe bowl, and heat the milk for thirty seconds. Stir in your nutmeg, and then pour it into the skillet. Cook uncovered for five minutes. Stir occasionally to keep from burning.

3. Get out a stockpot and cook your pasta per package instructions. Drain the pasta, and then save two tablespoons of pasta water.

4. Stir everything together, and add in the cheese and lemon juice and pasta water.

Nutrition

410 Calories

15g Protein

17g Fat

12g Carbohydrates

14. Asparagus Pasta

Difficulty: Professional level

Preparation Time: 8 minutes

Cooking Time: 33 minutes

Serving: 6

Size/ Portion: 2 ounces

Ingredients:

- 8 ounces farfalle pasta, uncooked
- 1 ½ cups asparagus
- 1-pint grape tomatoes, halved
- 2 tablespoons olive oil
- 2 cups mozzarella, fresh & drained
- 1/3 cup basil leaves, fresh & torn
- 2 tablespoons balsamic vinegar

Directions:

1. Start by heating the oven to 400, and then get out a stockpot. Cook your pasta per package instructions, and reserve ¼ cup of pasta water.

2. Get out a bowl and toss the tomatoes, oil, asparagus, and season with salt and pepper. Spread this mixture on a baking sheet, and bake for fifteen minutes. Stir twice in this time.

3. Remove your vegetables from the oven, and then add the cooked pasta to your baking sheet. Mix with a few tablespoons of pasta water so that your sauce becomes smoother.

4. Mix in your basil and mozzarella, drizzling with balsamic vinegar. Serve warm.

Nutrition:

307 Calories 18g Protein

14g Fat

5g Carbohydrates

15.   Feta & Spinach Pita Bake

Difficulty: Professional level

Time: 11 minutes

Cooking Time: 36 minutes

Serving: 6

Size/ Portion: 2 ounces

Ingredients:

- 2 roma tomatoes
- 6 whole wheat pita bread
- 1 jar sun dried tomato pesto
- 4 mushrooms, fresh & sliced
- 1 bunch spinach
- 2 tablespoons parmesan cheese
- 3 tablespoons olive oil
- ½ cup feta cheese

Directions:

1. Start by heating the oven to 350, and get to your pita bread. Spread the tomato pesto on the side of each one. Put them in a baking pan with the tomato side up.

2. Top with tomatoes, spinach, mushrooms, parmesan and feta. Drizzle with olive oil and season with pepper.

3. Bake for twelve minutes, and then serve cut into quarters.

Nutrition:

350 Calories

12g Protein

17g Fat

14g Carbohydrates

CHAPTER 6:

Side Dishes

1. Spring Sandwich

Difficulty: Novice level

Preparation Time: 10 minutes

Cooking Time: 25 minutes

Serving: 4

Size/ portion: 1 sandwich

Ingredients:

- 1 pinch of salt
- 1 pinch of black pepper
- 4 teaspoons of extra-virgin olive oil
- 4 eggs
- 4 multigrain sandwich thins
- 1 onion, finely diced
- 1 tomato, sliced thinly
- 2 cups of fresh baby spinach leaves
- 4 tablespoons of crumbled feta
- 1 sprig of fresh rosemary

Directions:

1.   Preheat your oven to 375 F.

2.   Slice the multigrain sandwich thins open and brush each side with one teaspoon of olive oil. Place them into the oven and toast for five minutes. Remove and set aside.

3.   Situate non-stick skillet over medium heat, add the remaining 2 teaspoons of olive oil and strip the leaves of rosemary off into the pan. Add in the eggs, one by one.

4.   Cook until the eggs have whitened, and the yolks stay runny. Flip once using a spatula and then remove from the heat.

5.   Place the multigrain thins onto serving plates, then place the spinach leaves on top, followed by sliced tomato, one egg, and a sprinkling of feta cheese. Add salt and pepper, then close your sandwich using the remaining multigrain thins.

Nutrition:

150 calories

15g fat

3g protein

5g Carbohydrates

2.   Lemon-Tahini Sauce

Difficulty: Professional level

Preparation Time:10 Minutes

Cooking Time:0 Minutes

Servings:1 Cup

Ingredients:

- ½ cup tahini
- One garlic clove, minced
- Juice and zest of 1 lemon
- ½ teaspoon salt, plus more as needed
- ½ cup warm water, plus more as needed

Directions:

1. Combine the tahini and garlic in a small bowl.
2. Add the lemon juice and zest, and salt to the bowl and stir to mix well.
3. Fold in the warm water and whisk until well combined and creamy. Feel free to

add more warm water if you like a thinner consistency.

4. Taste and add additional salt as needed.

5. Stock the sauce in a sealed vessel in the refrigerator for up to 5 days.

Nutrition:

Calories: 179 Fat: 15.5g

Protein: 5.1g

Carbs: 6.8g

Fiber: 3.0g

Sodium: 324mg

3. Springtime Quinoa Salad

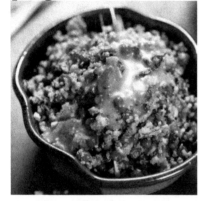

Difficulty: Novice level

Preparation Time: 10 minutes

Cooking Time: 25 minutes

Serving: 4

Size/ portion: 2 cups

Ingredients

For vinaigrette:

- 1 pinch of salt
- 1 pinch of black pepper
- ½ teaspoon of dried thyme
- ½ teaspoon of dried oregano
- ¼ cup of extra-virgin olive oil
- 1 tablespoon of honey
- juice of 1 lemon
- 1 clove of garlic, minced
- 2 tablespoons of fresh basil, diced

For salad:

- 1 ½ cups of cooked quinoa
- 4 cups of mixed leafy greens
- ½ cup of kalamata olives, halved and pitted
- ¼ cup of sun-dried tomatoes, diced
- ½ cup of almonds, raw, unsalted and diced

Directions:

1. Combine all the vinaigrette ingredients together, either by hand or using a blender or food processor. Set the vinaigrette aside in the refrigerator.

2. In a large salad bowl, combine the salad ingredients.

3. Drizzle the vinaigrette over the salad, then serve.

Nutrition:

201 calories 13g fat

4g protein 4g Carbohydrates

4. Spaghetti Niçoise

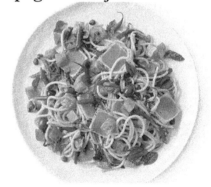

Difficulty: Novice level

Preparation Time: 15 minutes

Cooking Time: 20 minutes

Serving: 4

Size/ portion: 2 ounces

Ingredients

For pasta:

- 1 pinch of salt

- 1 pinch of black pepper
- ½ teaspoon of chili flakes
- 8 g of spaghetti
- 14 g of canned tuna chunks in oil
- 1/3 cup of kalamata olives
- 8 g of cherry tomatoes
- 3 g of arugula
- ½ cup of pine nuts

for dressing:

- 1 pinch of salt
- 1 pinch of black pepper
- 2 tablespoons of extra-virgin olive oil
- 1 tablespoon of Dijon mustard
- ¼ cup of lemon juice
- 1 tablespoon of lemon zest
- 1 clove of garlic, minced
- 1 tablespoon of capers

Directions:

1.　Stir all the ingredients for the dressing.

2.　Cook the pasta according the package instructions.

3.　Boil the eggs, deshell and cut them in half. Set this aside.

4.　Rinse and drain cooked pasta.

5.　Add the remaining ingredients, give it a toss, top with the eggs, and then drizzle with the mustard dressing.

Nutrition:

287 calories

14g fat

4g protein

3g Carbohydrates

5.　Tomato Poached Fish with Herbs and Chickpeas

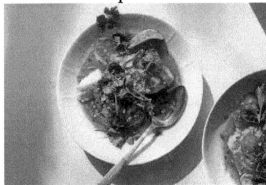

Difficulty: Novice level

Preparation Time: 20 minutes

Cooking Time: 20 minutes

Serving: 2

Size/ Portion: 1 lb.

Ingredients:

- 1 pinch of salt
- 1 pinch of black pepper
- 4 sprigs of fresh oregano
- 4 sprigs of fresh dill
- 1 ½ cups of water
- 1 cup of white wine
- 2 tablespoons of extra-virgin olive oil
- 1 tablespoon of tomato paste
- 2 cloves of garlic
- 2 shallots
- 1 lemon
- zest of 1 lemon
- 14 g can of chickpeas
- 8 g of cherry tomatoes
- 1 Fresno pepper
- 1 lb. of cod

Directions:

1.　Situate saucepan over high heat, cook olive oil, garlic, and shallots for two minutes.

2.   Add the salt, pepper, tomato paste, cherry tomatoes, chickpeas, and Fresno pepper.

3.   Stir in the water and wine. Place the fish into the center of the pan, ensuring it is submerged in the liquid. Sprinkle the lemon zest over the broth, then add the lemon slices and fresh herbs.

4.   Place a lid onto the saucepan and allow the broth to simmer for five to ten minutes, depending on the thickness of the cut of fish.

5.   When cooked, remove from the heat and serve over basmati rice. Top with a few toasted pistachios for added texture.

Nutrition:

351 calories 21g fat

9g protein 6g Carbohydrates

6.   Garlic Prawn and Pea Risotto

Difficulty: Novice level

Preparation Time: 15 minutes

Cooking Time: 30 minutes

Serving: 4

Size/ portion: 2 cups

Ingredients:

- 1 pinch of salt
- 1 pinch of black pepper
- 1 red chili
- 3 tablespoons of extra-virgin olive oil
- g of butter
- Juice of 1 lemon
- Zest of 1 lemon
- 50 Fl g of fish stock
- 1 cup of white wine
- 1 clove of garlic, finely diced
- 1 onion, diced
- 7 g of frozen peas
- 14 g of raw prawns
- g of Arborio rice

Directions:

1.   Rinse the prawns under running water and then remove their heads and shells. Keep these aside and keep the prawn meat aside.

2.   Situate saucepan over medium heat, add one tablespoon of olive oil, garlic, half of the finely diced chili, prawn heads, and shells. Cook until the shells change color. Boil stock, then turn the heat down to a simmer.

3.   In a separate medium saucepan over medium heat, add half the butter and the onions. Cook until the onions have softened. Add the risotto into the pan and stir continuously until you notice that the rice has become transparent in appearance.

4.   Stir wine to the rice and cook

5.   Begin to ladle the stock over the rice, one spoonful at a time. Ensure that the ladle of stock has evaporated before continuing to add the next. Stir in the peas and prawns.

6.   Continue adding stock until the rice has reached an al dente texture, soft with a starchy center, around 20 to 30 minutes. Continue to cook until the prawn meat has changed color.

7.   Remove the risotto from the heat, then add the remaining chili, olive oil, and lemon juice.

8.   Top with salt, pepper, lemon zest and serve.

Nutrition:

341 calories

16g fat

7g protein

5g Carbohydrates

7. Mediterranean Tostadas

Difficulty: Novice level

Preparation Time: 15 minutes

Cooking Time: 10 minutes

Serving: 4

Size/ portion: 1 tostada

Ingredients:

- 1 pinch salt
- 1 pinch black pepper
- 1 pinch oregano
- 1 pinch garlic powder
- 4 tostadas
- 1 tablespoon of extra-virgin olive oil
- ½ cup of milk
- ½ cup of roasted red pepper hummus
- 8 eggs, beaten
- ½ cup of green onion, finely diced
- ½ cup of red bell peppers, finely diced
- ½ cup of diced cucumber
- ½ cup of diced tomato
- ¼ cup of crumbled feta
- 1 handful of fresh basil

Directions:

1. Position non-stick skillet over medium heat, cook olive oil and red peppers. Cook until these have softened, then add the salt, pepper, oregano, garlic powder, milk, eggs, and onion.

2. Gently stir the mixture until you reach a scrambled egg consistency.

3. Once cooked through, remove from the heat.

4. Place a tostada onto each place, and top with the hummus, egg, tomato, cucumber, feta, and fresh basil leaves.

Nutrition: 251 calories 19g fat

6g protein 4g Carbohydrates

8. Vegetable Ratatouille

Difficulty: Novice level

Preparation Time: 15 minutes

Cooking Time: 40 minutes

Serving: 8

Size/ portion: 2 ounces

Ingredients:

- 1 pinch salt
- 1 pinch black pepper
- 1 pinch brown sugar
- ¼ cup extra-virgin olive oil
- ¼ cup of white wine
- 3 cloves of garlic
- 1 onion, diced
- 1 lb. of eggplant
- 1 cup of zucchini
- 1 ½ cups of canned tomato
- 1 red bell pepper, diced
- 1 green bell pepper, diced
- ½ cup of fresh basil

Directions:

1. Place saucepan over medium heat, cook olive oil and finely diced garlic and onion.

2. Add the cubed eggplant and continue to cook for a further 5 minutes.

3. Add the salt, pepper, and diced bell peppers. Allow to cook for another 3 minutes.

4. Add the sliced zucchini to the saucepan and cook for 3 minutes.

5. Mix white wine and canned tomatoes.

6. Allow to simmer for another five minutes. Taste the ratatouille.

7. Pull away from the heat, add the basil, and serve with a side portion of barley or brown rice.

Nutrition:

401 calories

19g fat

7g protein

8g Carbohydrates

9. Mixed Berry Pancakes and Ricotta

Difficulty: Novice level

Preparation Time: 15 minutes

Cooking Time: 25 minutes

Serving: 4

Size/ Portion: 2 pancakes

Ingredients:

- 1 pinch of salt
- ½ cup of milk
- 1 tablespoon of canola oil
- 2 eggs
- 1 ½ tablespoon of coarse brown sugar
- 1 teaspoon of baking powder
- ¼ teaspoon of baking soda
- 1 1/3 cup of all-purpose flour
- ½ cup of ricotta cheese
- 1 cup of mixed berries

Directions:

1. In a mixing bowl, combine the salt, sugar, baking powder, baking soda, and flour.

2. In a separate mixing bowl, combine the ricotta, eggs, oil, and milk.

3. Combine the wet mixture with the dry mixture. Mix well. Put aside for 10 minutes.

4. Place a large, non-stick frying pan over medium heat. When the pan is hot to the touch, spoon even amounts of the batter into the pan, making sure that the batter dollops do not touch.

5. When they begin to bubble through, flip them over and cook for a further minute or two.

6. Follow this process until all the batter has been made into pancakes.

7. Evenly divide the pancakes between four plates. Top with mixed berries and drizzle with maple syrup and a few extra dollops of ricotta.

Nutrition:

281 calories

19g fat

5g protein

11g Carbohydrates

10. Mediterranean Frittata

Difficulty: Novice level

Preparation Time: 5 minutes

Cooking Time: 25 minutes

Serving: 4

Size/ Portion: 1 Frittata

Ingredients:

- 1 pinch of salt
- 1 pinch of black pepper
- 1 tablespoon of extra-virgin olive oil
- 2 egg whites
- 6 eggs
- 1 cup of goat cheese
- 1 cup of Parmesan, shredded
- 8 g of mixed mushrooms
- 1 leek, diced
- 1 lb. of asparagus, finely sliced
- ½ cup of fresh basil leaves

Directions:

1. Preheat your oven to 400 F.

2. Scourge egg whites and eggs, salt, pepper, Parmesan cheese, and basil leaves. Set this aside.

3. In a large skillet, preferably non-stick, add the olive oil and leeks over medium heat. Cook until the leeks have softened, then add in the mushrooms, asparagus, and stir to combine and cook for a further 5 minutes.

4. Put egg mixture to the skillet, using a spatula to spread the eggs evenly over the mixture. Allow to cook for two minutes and then top with the goat cheese.

5. Place the skillet into the oven and allow to bake for five minutes

6. Remove from the oven and serve.

Nutrition:

317 calories

11g fat

3g protein

12g Carbohydrates

11. Caponata

Difficulty: Novice level

Preparation Time: 30 minutes

Cooking Time: 70 minutes

Serving: 6

Size/ Portion: 2 cups

Ingredients

For Caponata:

- 1 pinch of salt
- 1 pinch of black pepper
- Fl g of extra-virgin olive oil
- Fl g of red wine vinegar
- 2 shallots, diced
- 4 sticks of celery, diced
- 4 plum tomatoes, diced
- 3 eggplants
- 2 teaspoons of capers
- g of raisins
- ½ cup of pine nuts, raw
- ½ cup of fresh basil leaves

For bruschetta:

- Extra-virgin olive oil
- 1 clove of garlic
- 8 slices of ciabatta

Directions:

1. Place casserole over medium heat, cook olive oil and cubed eggplant

2. Remove the eggplant and set aside.

3. Add the diced shallots to the casserole and cook until softened. Follow by adding the plum tomatoes.

4. Allow the tomatoes to break down and return the eggplant cubes to this mixture.

5. Add the salt, pepper, vinegar, celery, capers, and raisins.

6. Set heat to low, cover and simmer for 40 minutes. Once the vegetables have cooked through, remove from the heat and set aside.

7. Coat the sliced ciabatta with olive oil and place onto a griddle pan over medium heat. Remove once charred on both sides. Rub the ciabatta slices with garlic cloves to enhance their flavor.

8. Top the caponata with the pine nuts and basil leaves, and serve with the sliced ciabatta on the side.

Nutrition:

311 calories

12g fat

2g protein

8g Carbohydrates

12. Fresh Deli Pasta

Difficulty: Novice level

Preparation Time: 15 minutes

Cooking Time: 30 minutes

Serving: 4

Size/ Portion: 2 ounces

Ingredients:

- 1 pinch of salt
- 1 pinch of black pepper
- 2 tablespoons of extra-virgin olive oil
- 2 teaspoons of white wine vinegar
- 1 clove of garlic
- 1 tomato, diced
- 10 sun-dried tomatoes
- 7 g of frozen peas
- g of pasta of your choice
- g of prosciutto
- ½ cup of fresh basil leaves

Directions:

1. In a large saucepan, cover the pasta with water and add a pinch of salt. Bring to a boil and allow to cook for 10 minutes, then add the frozen peas and cook for another 2 minutes.

2. Once the pasta is tender, drain it by placing it into a colander and running cold water over it. Give the colander a few shakes and set aside.

3. Pulse salt, pepper, olive oil, vinegar, garlic, 10 leaves of basil, tomato, and 5 of the sun-dried tomatoes into a blender.

4. Add the cooked pasta and peas to the serving bowl, add the remaining basil leaves, and lightly tear the prosciutto over the pasta.

5. Toss then serve.

Nutrition:

341 calories

11g fat

3g protein

9g Carbohydrates

13. Pistachio Arugula Salad

Difficulty: Novice level

Preparation Time: 20 minutes

Cooking Time: 0 minute

Serving: 6

Size/ Portion: 2 cups

Ingredients:

- ¼ cup olive oil
- 6 cups kale, chopped rough
- 2 cups arugula
- ½ teaspoon smoked paprika
- 2 tablespoons lemon juice, fresh
- 1/3 cup pistachios, unsalted & shelled
- 6 tablespoons parmesan, grated

Directions:

1. Get out a large bowl and combine your oil, lemon juice, kale and smoked paprika. Massage it into the leaves for about fifteen seconds. You then need to allow it to sit for ten minutes.

2. Mix everything together before serving with grated cheese on top.

Nutrition:

150 Calories

5g Protein

12g Fat

5g Carbohydrates

14. Potato Salad

Difficulty: Novice level

Preparation Time: 9 minutes

Cooking Time: 13 minutes

Serving: 6

Size/ Portion: 2 cups

Ingredients:

- 2 lbs. golden potatoes
- 3 tablespoons olive oil
- 3 tablespoons lemon juice, fresh
- 1 tablespoon olive brine
- ¼ teaspoon sea salt, fine
- ½ cup olives, sliced
- 1 cup celery, sliced
- 2 tablespoons oregano
- 2 tablespoons mint leaves

Directions:

1. Boil potatoes in saucepan before turning the heat down to medium-low. Cook for fifteen more minutes.
2. Get out a small bowl and whisk your oil, lemon juice, olive brine and salt together.
3. Drain your potatoes using a colander and transfer it to a serving bowl. Pour in three tablespoons of dressing over your potatoes, and mix well with oregano, and min along with the remaining dressing.

Nutrition: 175 Calories 3g Protein

7g Fat 8g Carbohydrates

15. Raisin Rice Pilaf

Difficulty: Novice level

Preparation Time: 13 minutes

Cooking Time: 8 minutes

Serving: 5

Size/ Portion: 2 cups

Ingredients:

- 1 tablespoon olive oil
- 1 teaspoon cumin
- 1 cup onion, chopped
- ½ cup carrot, shredded
- ½ teaspoon cinnamon
- 2 cups instant brown rice
- 1 ¾ cup orange juice
- 1 cup golden raisins
- ¼ cup water
- ½ cup pistachios, shelled
- fresh chives, chopped for garnish

Directions:

1. Place a medium saucepan over medium-high heat before adding in your oil. Add n your onion, and stir often so it doesn't burn. Cook for about five minutes and then add in your cumin, cinnamon and carrot. Cook for about another minute.
2. Add in your orange juice, water and rice. Boil before covering your saucepan. Turn the heat down to medium-low and then allow it to simmer for six to seven minutes.
3. Stir in your pistachios, chives and raisins. Serve warm.

Nutrition:

320 Calories 6g Protein

7g Fat 7g Carbohydrates

16. Lebanese Delight

Difficulty: Novice level

Preparation Time: 7 minutes

Cooking Time: 25 minutes

Serving: 5

Size/ Portion: 2 ounces

Ingredients:

- 1 tablespoon olive oil

- 1 cup vermicelli
- 3 cups cabbage, shredded
- 3 cups vegetable broth, low sodium
- ½ cup water
- 1 cup instant brown rice
- ¼ teaspoon sea salt, fine
- 2 cloves garlic
- ¼ teaspoon crushed red pepper
- ½ cup cilantro fresh & chopped
- lemon slices to garnish

Directions:

1. Get out a saucepan and then place it over medium-high heat. Add in your oil and once it's hot you will need to add in your pasta. Cook for three minutes or until your pasta is toasted. You will have to stir often in order to keep it from burning.

2. Ad in your cabbage, cooking for another four minutes. Continue to stir often.

3. Add in your water and rice. Season with salt, red pepper and garlic before bringing it all to a boil over high heat. Stir, and then cover. Once it's covered turn the heat down to medium-low. Allow it all to simmer for ten minutes.

4. Remove the pan from the burner and then allow it to sit without lifting the lid for five minutes. Take the garlic cloves out and then mash them using a fork. Place them back in, and stir them into the rice. Stir in your cilantro as well and serve warm. Garnish with lemon wedges if desired.

Nutrition:

259 Calories

7g Protein

4g Fat

8g Carbohydrates

17.   Mediterranean Sweet Potato

Difficulty: Novice level

Preparation Time: 6 minutes

Cooking Time: 25 minutes

Serving: 4

Size/ Portion: 1 cup

Ingredients:

- 4 sweet potatoes
- 15 ounce can chickpeas, rinsed & drained
- ½ tablespoon olive oil
- ½ teaspoon cumin
- ½ teaspoon coriander
- ½ teaspoon cinnamon
- 1 pinch sea salt, fine
- ½ teaspoon paprika
- ¼ cup hummus
- 1 tablespoon lemon juice, fresh
- 2-3 teaspoon dill, fresh
- 3 cloves garlic, minced
- unsweetened almond milk as needed

Directions:

1. Set oven to 400, and then get out a baking sheet. Line it with foil.

2. Wash your sweet potatoes before halving them lengthwise.

3. Take your olive oil, cumin, chickpeas, coriander, sea salt and paprika on your baking sheet. Rub the sweet potatoes with olive oil, placing them face down over the mixture.

4. Roast for twenty to twenty-five minutes.

5. Mix your dill, lemon juice, hummus, garlic and a dash of almond milk.

6. Smash the insides of the sweet potato down, topping with chickpea mixture and sauce before serving.

Nutrition: 313 Calories 8.6g Protein

9g fats 8g Carbohydrates

18. Flavorful Braised Kale

Difficulty: Novice level

Preparation Time: 7 minutes

Cooking Time: 32 minutes

Serving: 6

Size/ Portion: 1 cup

Ingredients:

- 1 lb. Kale
- 1 Cup Cherry Tomatoes, Halved
- 2 Teaspoons Olive Oil
- 4 Cloves Garlic, Sliced Thin
- ½ Cup Vegetable Stock
- ¼ Teaspoon Sea Salt, Fine
- 1 Tablespoon Lemon Juice, Fresh
- 1/8 Teaspoon Black Pepper

Directions:

1. Preheat olive oil in a frying pan using medium heat, and add in your garlic. Sauté for a minute or two until lightly golden.
2. Mix your kale and vegetable stock with your garlic, adding it to your pan.
3. Cover the pan and then turn the heat down to medium-low.
4. Allow it to cook until your kale wilts and part of your vegetable stock should be dissolved.
5. Stir in your tomatoes and cook without a lid until your kale is tender, and then remove it from heat.
6. Mix in your salt, pepper and lemon juice before serving warm.

Nutrition:

70 Calories

4g Protein

0.5g Fat

5g Carbohydrates

19. Bean Salad

Difficulty: Intermediate level

Preparation Time: 16 minutes

Cooking Time: 0 minutes

Serving: 6

Size/ Portion: 2 ounces

Ingredients:

- 1 can garbanzo beans, rinsed & drained
- 2 tablespoons balsamic vinegar
- ¼ cup olive oil
- 4 cloves garlic, chopped fine
- 1/3 cup parsley, fresh & chopped
- ¼ cup olive oil
- 1 red onion, diced
- 6 lettuce leaves
- ½ cup celery, chopped fine/black pepper to taste

Directions:

1. Make the vinaigrette dressing by whipping together your garlic, parsley, vinegar and pepper in a bowl.
2. Add the olive oil to this mixture and whisk before setting it aside.
3. Add in your onion and beans, and then pour your dressing on top. Toss then cover it. Chill before serving
4. Place a lettuce leaf on the plate when serving and spoon the mixture in. garnish with celery.

Nutrition:

218 Calories

7g Protein

0.1g Fat

3g Carbohydrates

20. Basil Tomato Skewers

Difficulty: Intermediate level

Preparation Time: 14 minutes

Cooking Time: 0 minute

Serving: 2

Size/ Portion: 1 skewer

Ingredients:

- 16 mozzarella balls, fresh & small
- 16 basil leaves, fresh
- 16 cherry tomatoes
- olive oil to drizzle
- sea salt & black pepper to taste

Directions:

1. Start by threading your basil, cheese and tomatoes together on small skewers.
2. Drizzle with oil before seasoning. Serve.

Nutrition:

46 Calories

7.6g Protein

0.9g Fat

8g Carbohydrates

21. Olives with Feta

Difficulty: Intermediate level

Preparation Time: 5 minutes

Cooking Time: 0 minute

Serving: 4

Size/ Portion: 1

Ingredients:

- ½ Cup Feta Cheese
- 1 Cup Kalamata Olives
- 2 Cloves Garlic, Sliced
- 2 Tablespoons Olive Oil
- 1 Lemon, Zested & Juiced
- 1 Teaspoon Rosemary, Fresh & Chopped

- Crushed Red Pepper
- Black Pepper to Taste

Directions:

1. Mix everything together and serve over crackers.

Nutrition:

71 Calories

4g Protein

2.6g Fat

9g Carbohydrates

22. Black Bean Medley

Difficulty: Intermediate level

Preparation Time: 5 minutes

Cooking Time: 0 minute

Serving: 4

Size/ Portion: 1 cup

Ingredients:

- 4 plum tomatoes, chopped
- 14.5 ounces black beans, canned & drained
- ½ red onion, sliced
- ¼ cup dill, fresh & chopped
- 1 lemon, juiced
- 2 tablespoons olive oil
- ¼ cup feta cheese, crumbled
- sea salt to taste

Directions:

1. Mix everything in a bowl except for your feta and salt. Top the beans with salt and feta.

Nutrition:

121 Calories

6g Protein

5g Fat

9g Carbohydrates

23. Chili Veggie Mix

Difficulty: Intermediate level

Preparation Time: 30 Minutes

Cooking Time: 3 Hours

Servings: 6

Ingredients:

- 1 cup cauliflower, chopped
- 1 cup broccoli, chopped
- 1 cup green peas
- 4 g asparagus, chopped
- One teaspoon salt
- One tablespoon lemon juice
- One teaspoon avocado oil
- ½ teaspoon chili flakes
- 2 cups water for the steamer

Directions:

1. Pour water into the pan and wait for it to boil.
2. Insert the steamer in the saucepan.
3. After this, place the vegetables in the steamer and close the lid.
4. Cook the vegetables for 10 minutes or until they are tender.
5. Then transfer the cooked vegetables to the mixing bowl.
6. In the shallow bowl, whisk together salt, lemon juice, avocado oil, and chili flakes.
7. Sprinkle the cooked vegetables with oil mixture and shake well.
8. Transfer the meat to the serving plates.

Nutrition:

Calories 34 Fat 0.3

Fiber 2.5 Carbs 6.2 Protein 2.5

24. Sautéed Collard Greens

Difficulty: Intermediate level

Preparation Time: 5 Minutes

Cooking Time: 45 Minutes

Servings: 6

Ingredients:

- 1-pound fresh collard greens, cut into 2-inch pieces
- One pinch of red pepper flakes
- 3 cups chicken broth
- One teaspoon pepper
- One teaspoon salt
- Two cloves garlic, minced
- One large onion, chopped
- Three slices of bacon
- One tablespoon olive oil

Directions:

1. Using a large skillet, heat oil on medium-high heat. Sauté bacon until crisp. Remove it from the pan and crumble it once cooled. Set it aside.
2. Using the same pan, sauté onion, and cook until tender. Add garlic until aromatic. Put the collard greens and cook until they start to wilt.
3. Pour in the chicken broth and season with pepper, salt, and red pepper flakes. Lessen the heat to low, then simmer for 45 minutes.

Nutrition:

Calories per **Serving:** 20

Carbs: 3.0g

Protein: 1.0g

Fat: 1.0g

25. Garlic Basil Zucchini

Difficulty: Intermediate level

Preparation Time: 5 Minutes

Cooking Time: 8 Minutes

Servings: 4

Ingredients:

- 14 g zucchini, sliced
- 1/4 cup fresh basil, chopped
- 1/2 tsp red pepper flakes
- 14 g can tomato, chopped
- 1 tsp garlic, minced
- 1/2 onion, chopped
- 1/4 cup feta cheese, crumbled
- 1 tbsp. olive oil
- Salt

Directions:

1. Add oil into the inner pot of the instant pot and set the pot on sauté mode.
2. Add onion and garlic and sauté for minutes.
3. Add remaining ingredients except for feta cheese and stir well.
4. Seal pot with lid and cook on high for 6 minutes.
5. Once done, allow to release pressure naturally. Remove lid.
6. Top with feta cheese and serve.

Nutrition:

Calories 99

Fat 5.7 g

Carbohydrates 10.4 g

Sugar 6.1 g

Protein 3.7 g

Cholesterol 8 mg

CHAPTER 7:

Appetizer and Snack Recipes

1. Marinated Feta and Artichokes

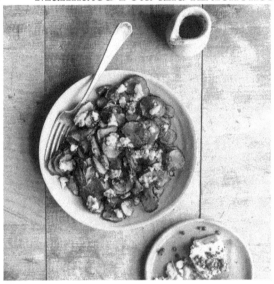

Difficulty: Novice level

Preparation Time: 10 minutes + 4 hours

Cooking Time: 0 minute

Serving: 3

Size/ Portion: 1/3 cup

Ingredients:

- 4 ounces traditional Greek feta, cut into ½-inch cubes

- 4 ounces drained artichoke hearts, quartered lengthwise

- 1/3 cup extra-virgin olive oil

- Zest and juice of 1 lemon

- 2 tablespoons roughly chopped fresh rosemary

- 2 tablespoons roughly chopped fresh parsley

- ½ teaspoon black peppercorns

Direction

1. In a glass bowl, combine the feta and artichoke hearts. Add the olive oil, lemon zest and juice, rosemary, parsley, and peppercorns and toss gently to coat, being sure not to crumble the feta.

2. Cover and chill for 4 hours before serving.

Nutrition:

235 Calories

23g Fat

4g Protein

11g Carbohydrates

2. Citrus-Marinated Olives

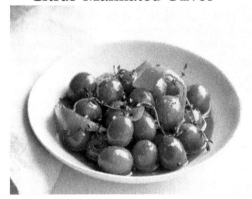

Difficulty: Novice level

Preparation Time: 10 minutes + 4 hours

Cooking Time: 0 minute

Serving: 4

Size/ Portion: ¼ cup

Ingredients:

- 2 cups mixed green olives with pits

- ¼ cup red wine vinegar

- ¼ cup extra-virgin olive oil
- 4 garlic cloves, finely minced
- Zest and juice orange
- 1 teaspoon red pepper flakes
- 2 bay leaves
- ½ teaspoon ground cumin
- ½ teaspoon ground allspice

Direction:

1. In a jar, mix olives, vinegar, oil, garlic, orange zest and juice, red pepper flakes, bay leaves, cumin, and allspice. Cover and chill for 4 hours, tossing again before serving.

Nutrition:

133 Calories 14g Fat

1g Protein 4g Carbohydrates

3. Olive Tapenade with Anchovies

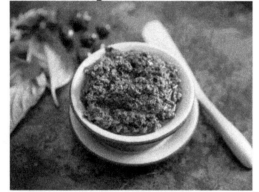

Difficulty: Novice level

Preparation Time: 70 minutes

Cooking Time: 0 minute

Serving: 4

Size/ Portion: 1/3 cup

Ingredient:

- 2 cups pitted Kalamata olives
- 2 anchovy fillets
- 2 teaspoons capers
- 1 garlic clove

- 1 cooked egg yolk
- 1 teaspoon Dijon mustard
- ¼ cup extra-virgin olive oil

Direction:

1. Wash olives in cold water and drain well.

2. In a food processor, mix drained olives, anchovies, capers, garlic, egg yolk, and Dijon.With the food processor running, slowly stream in the olive oil.

3. Wrap and refrigerate at least 1 hour. Serve with Seedy Crackers.

Nutrition: 179 Calories 19g Fat

2g Protein 12g Carbohydrates

4. Greek Deviled Eggs

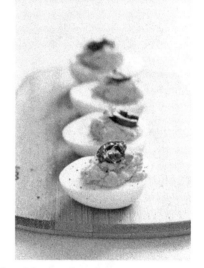

Difficulty: Novice level

Preparation Time: 45 minutes

Cooking Time: 15 minutes

Serving: 4

Size/ Portion: 1 piece

Ingredients:

- 4 large hardboiled eggs
- 2 tablespoons Roasted Garlic Aioli
- ½ cup feta cheese
- 8 pitted Kalamata olives

- 2 tablespoons chopped sun-dried tomatoes
- 1 tablespoon minced red onion
- ½ teaspoon dried dill
- ¼ teaspoon black pepper

Direction:

1. Slice the hardboiled eggs in half lengthwise, remove the yolks, and place the yolks in a medium bowl. Reserve the egg white halves and set aside. Smash the yolks well with a fork. Add the aioli, feta, olives, sun-dried tomatoes, onion, dill, and pepper and stir to combine until smooth and creamy.

2. Spoon the filling into each egg white half and chill for 30 minutes, or up to 24 hours, covered.

Nutrition: 147 Calories 11g Fat

9g Protein 8g Carbohydrates

5. Manchego Crackers

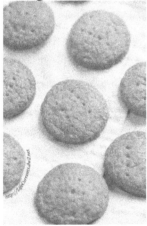

Difficulty: Novice level

Preparation Time: 55 minutes

Cooking Time: 15 minutes

Serving: 4

Size/ Portion: 10 pieces

Ingredients:

- 4 tablespoons butter, at room temperature

- 1 cup Manchego cheese
- 1 cup almond flour
- 1 teaspoon salt, divided
- ¼ teaspoon black pepper
- 1 large egg

Direction:

1. Using an electric mixer, scourge butter and shredded cheese.

2. Mix almond flour with ½ teaspoon salt and pepper. Mix almond flour mixture to the cheese, mixing constantly to form a ball.

3. Situate onto plastic wrap and roll into a cylinder log about 1½ inches thick. Wrap tightly and refrigerate for at least 1 hour.

4. Preheat the oven to 350°F. Prep two baking sheets with parchment papers.

5. For egg wash, blend egg and remaining ½ teaspoon salt.

6. Slice the refrigerated dough into small rounds, about ¼ inch thick, and place on the lined baking sheets.

7. Egg wash the tops of the crackers and bake for 15 minutes. Pull out from the oven and situate in wire rack.

8. Serve.

Nutrition:

243 Calories 23g Fat

8g Protein 4g Carbohydrates

6. Burrata Caprese Stack

Difficulty: Intermediate level

Preparation Time: 5 minutes

Cooking Time: 0 minutes

Serving: 4

Size/ Portion: 1 stack

Ingredients:

- 1 large organic tomato
- ½ teaspoon salt

- ¼ teaspoon black pepper
- 1 (4-ounce) ball burrata cheese
- 8 fresh basil leaves
- 2 tablespoons extra-virgin olive oil
- 1 tablespoon red wine

Direction

1. Slice the tomato into 4 thick slices, removing any tough center core and sprinkle with salt and pepper. Place the tomatoes, seasoned-side up, on a plate.

2. On a separate rimmed plate, slice the burrata into 4 thick slices and place one slice on top of each tomato slice. Top each with one-quarter of the basil and pour any reserved burrata cream from the rimmed plate over top.

3. Drizzle with olive oil and vinegar and serve with a fork and knife.

Nutrition:

153 Calories

13g Fat

7g Protein

6g Carbohydrates

7. Zucchini-Ricotta Fritters with Lemon-Garlic Aioli

Difficulty: Intermediate level

Preparation Time: 30 minutes

Cooking Time: 25 minutes

Serving: 4

Size/ Portion: 1 fritter

Ingredient:

- 1 large zucchini
- 1 teaspoon salt, divided
- ½ cup whole-milk ricotta cheese
- 2 scallions
- 1 large egg
- 2 garlic cloves

- 2 tablespoons fresh mint (optional)
- 2 teaspoons grated lemon zest
- ¼ teaspoon freshly ground black pepper
- ½ cup almond flour
- 1 teaspoon baking powder
- 8 tablespoons extra-virgin olive oil
- 8 tablespoons Roasted Garlic Aioli

Direction

1. Place the shredded zucchini in a colander or on several layers of paper towels. Sprinkle with ½ teaspoon salt and let sit for 10 minutes. Using another layer of paper towel, press down on the zucchini to release any excess moisture and pat dry.

2. In a large bowl, combine the drained zucchini, ricotta, scallions, egg, garlic, mint (if using), lemon zest, remaining ½ teaspoon salt, and pepper and stir well.

3. Blend almond flour and baking powder. Mix in flour mixture into the zucchini mixture and let rest for 10 minutes.

4. In a large skillet, working in four batches, fry the fritters. For each batch of four, heat 2 tablespoons olive oil over medium-high heat. Add 1 heaping tablespoon of zucchini batter per fritter, pressing down with the back of a spoon to form 2- to 3-inch fritters. Cover and let fry 2 minutes before flipping. Fry another 2 to 3 minutes, covered.

5. Repeat for the remaining three batches, using 2 tablespoons of the olive oil for each batch.

6. Serve with aioli.

Nutrition:

448 Calories

42g Fat

8g Protein

8g Carbohydrates

8. Salmon-Stuffed Cucumbers

Difficulty: Intermediate level

Preparation Time: 10 minutes

Cooking Time: 0 minute

Serving: 4

Size/ Portion: 1 piece

Ingredients:

- 2 large cucumbers, peeled
- 1 (4-ounce) can red salmon
- 1 medium very ripe avocado
- 1 tablespoon extra-virgin olive oil
- Zest and juice of 1 lime
- 3 tablespoons chopped fresh cilantro
- ½ teaspoon salt
- ¼ teaspoon black pepper

Direction:

1. Slice the cucumber into 1-inch-thick segments and using a spoon, scrape seeds out of center of each segment and stand up on a plate.
2. In a medium bowl, mix salmon, avocado, olive oil, lime zest and juice, cilantro, salt, and pepper.
3. Spoon the salmon mixture into the center of each cucumber segment and serve chilled.

Nutrition:

159 Calories 11g Fat

9g Protein 20g Carbohydrates

9. Sfougato

Difficulty: Intermediate level

Preparation Time: 9 minutes

Cooking Time: 13 minutes

Serving: 4

Size/ Portion: 2 tablespoons

Ingredients:

- ½ cup crumbled feta cheese

- ¼ cup bread crumbs
- 1 medium onion
- 4 tablespoons all-purpose flour
- 2 tablespoons fresh mint
- ½ teaspoon salt
- ½ teaspoon ground black pepper
- 1 tablespoon dried thyme
- 6 large eggs, beaten
- 1 cup water

Direction:

1. In a medium bowl, mix cheese, bread crumbs, onion, flour, mint, salt, pepper, and thyme. Stir in eggs.
2. Spray an 8" round baking dish with nonstick cooking spray. Pour egg mixture into dish.
3. Place rack in the Instant Pot® and add water. Fold a long piece of foil in half lengthwise. Lay foil over rack to form a sling and top with dish. Cover loosely with foil. Seal lid, put steam release in Sealing, select Manual, and time to 8 minutes.
4. When the timer alarms, release the pressure. Uncover. Let stand 5 minutes, then remove dish from pot.

Nutrition:

274 Calories 14g Fat

17g Protein 13g Carbohydrates

10. Goat Cheese–Mackerel Pâté

Difficulty: Intermediate level

Preparation Time: 10 minutes

Cooking Time: 0 minute

Serving: 4

Size/ Portion: 1 piece

Ingredients:

- 4 ounces olive oil-packed wild-caught mackerel

- 2 ounces goat cheese
- Zest and juice of 1 lemon
- 2 tablespoons chopped fresh parsley
- 2 tablespoons chopped fresh arugula
- 1 tablespoon extra-virgin olive oil
- 2 teaspoons chopped capers
- 2 teaspoons fresh horseradish (optional)

Direction:

1. In a food processor, blender, or large bowl with immersion blender, combine the mackerel, goat cheese, lemon zest and juice, parsley, arugula, olive oil, capers, and horseradish (if using). Process or blend until smooth and creamy.
2. Serve with crackers, cucumber rounds, endive spears, or celery.

Nutrition:

118 Calories

8g Fat

9g Protein

15g Carbohydrates

11.   Baba Ghanoush

Difficulty: Intermediate level

Preparation Time: 9 minutes

Cooking Time: 11 minutes

Serving: 8

Size/ Portion: 3 tablespoons

Ingredients:

- 2 tablespoons extra-virgin olive oil
- 1 large eggplant
- 3 cloves garlic
- ½ cup water
- 3 tablespoons fresh flat-leaf parsley
- ½ teaspoon salt
- ¼ teaspoon smoked paprika

- 2 tablespoons lemon juice
- 2 tablespoons tahini

Direction

1. Press the Sauté button on the Instant Pot® and add 1 tablespoon oil. Add eggplant and cook until it begins to soften, about 5 minutes. Add garlic and cook 30 seconds.
2. Add water and close lid, click steam release to Sealing, select Manual, and time to 6 minutes. Once the timer rings, quick-release the pressure. Select Cancel and open lid.
3. Strain cooked eggplant and garlic and add to a food processor or blender along with parsley, salt, smoked paprika, lemon juice, and tahini. Add remaining 1 tablespoon oil and process. Serve warm or at room temperature.

Nutrition:

79 Calories

6g Fat

2g Protein

3g Carbohydrates

12.   Instant Pot® Salsa

Difficulty: Intermediate level

Preparation Time: 9 minutes

Cooking Time: 22 minutes

Serving: 12

Size/ Portion: 2 tablespoons

Ingredients:

- 12 cups seeded diced tomatoes
- 6 ounces tomato paste
- 2 medium yellow onions
- 6 small jalapeño peppers
- 4 cloves garlic
- ¼ cup white vinegar
- ¼ cup lime juice

- 2 tablespoons granulated sugar
- 2 teaspoons salt
- ¼ cup chopped fresh cilantro

Direction:

1. Place tomatoes, tomato paste, onions, jalapeños, garlic, vinegar, lime juice, sugar, and salt in the Instant Pot® and stir well. Close it, situate steam release to Sealing. Click Manual button, and time to 20 minutes.

2. Once timer beeps, quick-release the pressure. Open, stir in cilantro, and press the Cancel button.

3. Let salsa cool to room temperature, about 40 minutes, then transfer to a storage container and refrigerate overnight.

Nutrition:

68 Calories

0.1g Fat

2g Protein

5g Carbohydrates

13. Taste of the Mediterranean Fat Bombs

Difficulty: Intermediate level

Preparation Time: 15 minutes + 4 hours

Cooking Time: 0 minute

Serving: 6

Size/ Portion: 1 fat bomb

Ingredients:

- 1 cup crumbled goat cheese
- 4 tablespoons jarred pesto
- 12 pitted Kalamata olives
- ½ cup finely chopped walnuts
- 1 tablespoon chopped fresh rosemary

Direction:

1. Mix goat cheese, pesto, and olives. Cool for 4 hours to harden.

2. Create the mixture into 6 balls, about ¾-inch diameter. The mixture will be sticky.

3. In a small bowl, place the walnuts and rosemary and roll the goat cheese balls in the nut mixture to coat.

Nutrition

166 Calories

15g Fat

5g Protein

8g Carbohydrates

14. Cream of Cauliflower Gazpacho

Difficulty: Intermediate level

Preparation Time: 15 minutes

Cooking Time: 25 minutes

Serving: 6

Size/ Portion: 2 cups

Ingredients:

- 1 cup raw almonds
- ½ teaspoon salt
- ½ cup extra-virgin olive oil
- 1 small white onion
- 1 small head cauliflower
- 2 garlic cloves
- 2 cups chicken stock
- 1 tablespoon red wine vinegar
- ¼ teaspoon freshly ground black pepper

Direction:

1. Boil almonds to the water for 1 minute. Drain in a colander and run under cold water. Pat dry. Discard the skins.

2. In a food processor or blender, blend together the almonds and salt. With the processor running, drizzle in ½ cup extra-virgin olive oil, scraping down the sides as needed. Set the almond paste aside.

3. In a stockpot, cook remaining 1 tablespoon olive oil over medium-high

heat. Sauté onion for 4 minutes. Add the cauliflower florets and sauté for another 3 to 4 minutes. Cook garlic for 1 minute more.

4. Add 2 cups stock and bring to a boil. Cover, reduce the heat to medium-low, and simmer the vegetables until tender, 8 to 10 minutes. Pull out from the heat and allow to cool slightly.

5. Blend vinegar and pepper with an immersion blender. With the blender running, add the almond paste and blend until smooth, adding extra stock if the soup is too thick.

6. Serve warm, or chill in refrigerator at least 4 to 6 hours to serve a cold gazpacho.

Nutrition:

505 Calories

45g Fat

10g Protein

11g Carbohydrates

15.   Classic Hummus

Difficulty: Professional level

Preparation Time: 8 minutes

Cooking Time: 30 minutes

Serving: 6

Size/ Portion: 2 tablespoons

Ingredient:

- 1 cup dried chickpeas
- 4 cups water
- 1 tablespoon plus ¼ cup extra-virgin olive oil
- 1/3 cup tahini
- 1½ teaspoons ground cumin
- ¾ teaspoon salt
- ½ teaspoon ground black pepper
- ½ teaspoon ground coriander

- 1/3 cup lemon juice
- 1 teaspoon minced garlic

Direction:

1. Position chickpeas, water, and 1 tablespoon oil in the Instant Pot®. Close, select steam release to Sealing, click Manual, and time to 30 minutes.

2. When the timer rings, quick-release the pressure and open lid. Press the Cancel button and open lid. Drain, reserving the cooking liquid.

3. Blend chickpeas, remaining ¼ cup oil, tahini, cumin, salt, pepper, coriander, lemon juice, and garlic in a food processor. Serve.

Nutrition:

152 Calories

12g Fat

4g Protein

11g Carbohydrates

16.   Passion   Fruit   and   Spicy Couscous

Difficulty: Novice level

Preparation Time: 15 minutes

Cooking Time: 15 minutes

Serving: 4

Size/ portion: 1 cup

Ingredients:

- 1 pinch of salt
- 1 pinch of allspice
- 1 teaspoon of mixed spice
- 1 cup of boiling water
- 2 teaspoons of extra-virgin olive oil
- ½ cup of full-fat Greek yogurt
- ½ cup of honey
- 1 cup of couscous
- 1 teaspoon of orange zest

- 2 oranges, peeled and sliced
- 2 tablespoons of passion fruit pulp
- ½ cup of blueberries
- ½ cup of walnuts, roasted and unsalted
- 2 tablespoons of fresh mint

Directions:

1. In a mixing bowl, combine the salt, allspice, mixed spice, honey, couscous, and boiling water. Cover the bowl and allow to rest for five to ten minutes, or until the water has been absorbed. Using a fork, give the mixture a good stir, then add the diced walnuts.

2. In a separate bowl, combine the passion fruit, yogurt, and orange zest.

3. To serve, dish the couscous up into four bowls, add the yogurt mixture, and top with the sliced orange, blueberries, and mint leaves.

Nutrition:

100 calories

10.5g fat

2.1g protein

8.7g Carbohydrates

17. Honey and Vanilla Custard Cups with Crunchy Filo Pastry

Difficulty: Novice level

Preparation Time: 25 minutes

Cooking Time: 2 hours

Serving: 4

Size/ Portion: 2 cups

Ingredients:

- 1 vanilla bean, cut lengthways
- 2 cups of full-fat milk
- 1/3 cup of honey
- 1 tablespoon of brown sugar
- 2 tablespoons of custard powder

- 4 to 6 ripe figs, quartered
- 1 sheet of filo pastry
- 2 tablespoons of raw pistachios

Directions:

1. Situate saucepan over medium heat, simmer vanilla bean, milk, and honey

2. In a heatproof dish, combine the sugar and custard powder. Transfer the milk mixture into the bowl containing the custard powder. Using a whisk, combine well and then transfer back into the saucepan.

3. Bring to a boil, constantly whisking until the custard thickens. Remove the vanilla bean.

4. Pour the custard into cups and allow to chill in the refrigerator for 2 hours.

5. Heat your oven to 350 F and line a baking tray with parchment.

6. Put the pastry sheet onto an even surface and spray lightly with olive oil cooking spray.

7. Sprinkle half the pistachios over the pastry and then fold the pastry in half. Heat up 2 tablespoons of honey in the microwave, then coat the pastry.

8. Place the pastry into the oven and allow to bake for 10 minutes. Remove from heat and allow it to cool.

9. Gently break the filo pastry into pieces, then top the custard with the shards and fresh-cut figs.

Nutrition:

307 calories

17g fat

4g protein

6.5g Carbohydrates

18.   Citrus Cups

Difficulty: Novice level

Preparation Time: 15 minutes

Cooking Time: 15 minutes

Serving: 4

Size/ Portion: 2 cups

Ingredients:

- ½ cup of water
- 1 tablespoon of orange juice
- 3 cups of full-fat Greek yogurt
- 1 vanilla bean
- 1 ruby grapefruit
- 2 mandarins
- 1 orange
- 6 strips of mandarin rind
- 1/3 cup of powdered sugar
- 1 small handful of fresh mint leaves

Directions:

1.   Slice open the vanilla bean lengthways and transfer the seeds into a medium saucepan. Add the pod to the saucepan as well, followed by the water, sugar, and mandarin rind.

2.   Bring the mixture to a boil, then turn down to a simmer and cook for five minutes or until the syrup has thickened.

3.   Allow to cool, remove the pod, and stir in the orange juice.

4.   Pour the syrup over the sliced citrus fruits and allow to rest.

5.   Dish the yogurt up into four bowls, top with the citrus and syrup, sprinkle with a bit of mint, then serve.

Nutrition:

217 calories

16g fat

4g protein

3.2g Carbohydrates

19.   Bananas Foster

Difficulty: Novice level

Preparation Time: 5 minutes

Cooking Time: 6 minutes

Servings: 4

Size/ Portion: 1 cup

Ingredients

- 2/3 cup dark brown sugar
- 1/4 cup butter
- 3 1/2 tablespoons rum
- 1 1/2 teaspoons vanilla extract
- 1/2 teaspoon of ground cinnamon
- 3 bananas, peeled and cut lengthwise and broad
- 1/4 cup coarsely chopped nuts
- vanilla ice cream

Direction

1.   Melt the butter in a deep-frying pan over medium heat. Stir in sugar, rum, vanilla, and cinnamon.

2.   When the mixture starts to bubble, place the bananas and nuts in the pan. Bake until the bananas are hot, 1 to 2 minutes. Serve immediately with vanilla ice cream.

Nutrition:

534 calories 23.8g fat

4.6g protein 5.7g Carbohydrates

20.   Cranberry Orange Cookies

Difficulty: Novice level

Preparation Time: 20 minutes

Cooking Time: 16 minutes

Servings: 24

Size/ Portion: 2 cookies

Ingredients

- 1 cup of soft butter
- 1 cup of white sugar

- 1/2 cup brown sugar
- 1 egg
- 1 teaspoon grated orange peel
- 2 tablespoons orange juice
- 2 1/2 cups flour
- 1/2 teaspoon baking powder
- 1/2 teaspoon salt
- 2 cups chopped cranberries
- 1/2 cup chopped walnuts (optional)

Icing:

- 1/2 teaspoon grated orange peel
- 3 tablespoons orange juice
- 1 ½ cup confectioner's sugar

Direction

1. Preheat the oven to 190 ° C.

2. Blend butter, white sugar, and brown sugar. Beat the egg until everything is well mixed. Mix 1 teaspoon of orange zest and 2 tablespoons of orange juice. Mix the flour, baking powder, and salt; stir in the orange mixture.

3. Mix the cranberries and, if used, the nuts until well distributed. Place the dough with a spoon on ungreased baking trays.

4. Bake in the preheated oven for 12 to 14 minutes. Cool on racks.

5. In a small bowl, mix icing ingredients. Spread over cooled cookies.

Nutrition:

110 calories

4.8g fat

1.1 g protein

2.3g Carbohydrates

CHAPTER 8:

Lunch and Dinner

Lunch and Dinner (Seafood Recipes)

1. Seafood Souvlaki Bowl

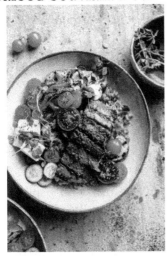

Difficulty: Novice level

Preparation Time: 20 minutes

Cooking Time: 20 minutes

Serving: 4

Size/ Portion: 2 cups

Ingredients

For salmon

- 1 pinch of salt
- 1 pinch of black pepper
- 1 tablespoon of fresh oregano
- 1 tablespoon of paprika
- 1 tablespoon of fresh dill
- 3 tablespoons of extra-virgin olive oil
- 2 tablespoons of balsamic vinegar
- 6 tablespoons of freshly squeezed lemon juice

- 2 cloves of garlic, minced
- 1 lb. of fresh salmon, cut into 4 fillets

Ingredients:

- 1 pinch of salt
- 1 pinch of black pepper
- 2 tablespoons of extra-virgin olive oil
- Juice of 1 lemon
- 2 red bell peppers, diced
- 1 large cucumber, diced
- 1 zucchini, sliced
- 1 cup of cherry tomatoes, halved
- ½ cup of kalamata olives, pitted and halved
- 1 cup of dry pearled couscous
- 8 g of feta, cubed

Directions:

1.   Cook the couscous following the package instructions and set aside.

2.   In a medium mixing bowl, add all the souvlaki ingredients apart from the fish. Combine well, then coat each fish fillet. Allow the fillets to rest in the bowl for 15 minutes.

3.   In a separate mixing bowl, combine the sliced bell peppers and zucchini. Add two tablespoons of olive oil, salt, and pepper. Combine and set aside.

4. In a medium skillet over medium heat, cook the salmon until tender, then remove from the heat.

5. Add the sliced peppers and zucchini to the skillet and cook for three minutes until you see charring, then remove from the heat.

6. To serve, dish the couscous up into four serving bowls and top with the lemon juice. Add the cooked salmon, charred vegetables, cucumber, tomatoes, olives, and feta.

Nutrition:

159 calories 11g fat

2g protein 3g Carbohydrates

2. Baked Cod with Vegetables

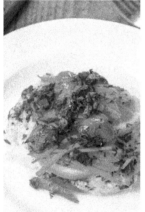

Difficulty: Novice level

Preparation Time: 15 minutes

Cooking Time: 25 minutes

Serving: 2

Size/ Portion: 2 pieces

Ingredients:

- 1 pound (454 g) thick cod fillet, cut into 4 even portions
- ¼ teaspoon onion powder (optional)
- ¼ teaspoon paprika
- 3 tablespoons extra-virgin olive oil
- 4 medium scallions
- ½ cup fresh chopped basil, divided
- 3 tablespoons minced garlic (optional)
- 2 teaspoons salt
- 2 teaspoons freshly ground black pepper
- ¼ teaspoon dry marjoram (optional)
- 6 sun-dried tomato slices
- ½ cup dry white wine
- ½ cup crumbled feta cheese
- 1 (15-ounce / 425-g) can oil-packed artichoke hearts, drained
- 1 lemon, sliced
- 1 cup pitted kalamata olives
- 1 teaspoon capers (optional)
- 4 small red potatoes, quartered

Direction:

1. Set oven to 375°F (190°C).

2. Season the fish with paprika and onion powder (if desired).

3. Heat an ovenproof skillet over medium heat and sear the top side of the cod for about 1 minute until golden. Set aside.

4. Heat the olive oil in the same skillet over medium heat. Add the scallions, ¼ cup of basil, garlic (if desired), salt, pepper, marjoram (if desired), tomato slices, and white wine and stir to combine. Boil then removes from heat.

5. Evenly spread the sauce on the bottom of skillet. Place the cod on top of the tomato basil sauce and scatter with feta cheese. Place the artichokes in the skillet and top with the lemon slices.

6. Scatter with the olives, capers (if desired), and the remaining ¼ cup of basil. Pullout from the heat and transfer to the preheated oven. Bake for 15 to 20 minutes

7. Meanwhile, place the quartered potatoes on a baking sheet or wrapped in

aluminum foil. Bake in the oven for 15 minutes.

8. Cool for 5 minutes before serving.

Nutrition:

1168 calories 60g fat 64g protein

5g Carbohydrates

3.   Tuna Croquettes

Difficulty: Novice level

Preparation Time: 40 minutes

Cooking Time: 25 minutes

Serving: 12

Size/ Portion: 3 pieces

Ingredients:

- 6 tablespoons extra-virgin olive oil, plus 1 to 2 cups

- 5 tablespoons almond flour, plus 1 cup, divided

- 1¼ cups heavy cream

- 1 (4-ounce) can olive oil-packed yellowfin tuna

- 1 tablespoon chopped red onion

- 2 teaspoons minced capers

- ½ teaspoon dried dill

- ¼ teaspoon freshly ground black pepper

- 2 large eggs

- 1 cup panko breadcrumbs

Direction

1. In a huge skillet, heat 6 tablespoons olive oil over medium-low heat. Add 5 tablespoons almond flour and cook, stirring constantly, until a smooth paste forms and the flour browns slightly, 2 to 3 minutes.

2. Increase the heat to medium-high and gradually add the heavy cream, whisking constantly for 5 minutes.

3. Pull out from heat and stir in the tuna, red onion, capers, dill, and pepper.

4. Pour into 8-inch square baking dish that is well coated with olive oil and allow to cool to room temperature. Cover and chill for 4 hours.

5. To form the croquettes, set out three bowls. In one, beat together the eggs. In another, add the remaining almond flour. In the third, add the panko. Line a baking sheet with parchment paper.

6. Situate a tablespoon of cold prepared dough into the flour mixture and roll to coat. Shake off excess and, using your hands, roll into an oval.

7. Dip the croquette into the beaten egg, then lightly coat in panko. Set on lined baking sheet and repeat with the remaining dough.

8. In a small saucepan, cook 1 to 2 cups of olive oil over medium-high heat.

9. Once the oil is heated, fry the croquettes 3 or 4 at a time.

Nutrition:

245 Calories 22g Fat 6g Protein

8g Carbohydrates

4.   Smoked Salmon Crudités

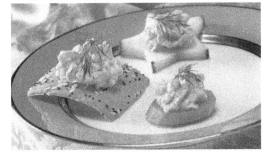

Difficulty: Novice level

Preparation Time: 10 minutes

Cooking Time: 0 minute

Serving: 4

Size/ Portion: 1 piece

Ingredients:

- 6 ounces smoked wild salmon

- 2 tablespoons Roasted Garlic Aioli

- 1 tablespoon Dijon mustard
- 1 tablespoon chopped scallions
- 2 teaspoons chopped capers
- ½ teaspoon dried dill
- 4 endive spears or hearts of romaine
- ½ English cucumber

Direction:

1. Cut the smoked salmon. Add the aioli, Dijon, scallions, capers, and dill and mix well.
2. Top endive spears and cucumber rounds with a spoonful of smoked salmon mixture and enjoy chilled.

Nutrition:

92 Calories

5g Fat

9g Protein

7g Carbohydrates

5. Slow Cooker Salmon in Foil

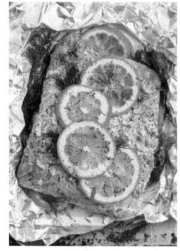

Difficulty: Novice level

Preparation Time: 5 minutes

Cooking Time: 2 hours

Serving: 2

Size/ Portion: 6 ounces

Ingredients:

- 2 (6-ounce / 170-g) salmon fillets

- 1 tablespoon olive oil
- 2 cloves garlic, minced
- ½ tablespoon lime juice
- 1 teaspoon finely chopped fresh parsley
- ¼ teaspoon black pepper

Direction

1. Spread a length of foil onto a work surface and place the salmon fillets in the middle.
2. Blend olive oil, garlic, lime juice, parsley, and black pepper. Brush the mixture over the fillets. Fold the foil over and crimp the sides to make a packet.
3. Place the packet into the slow cooker, cover, and cook on High for 2 hours
4. Serve hot.

Nutrition:

446 calories

21g fat

65g protein

25g Carbohydrates

6. Dill Chutney Salmon

Difficulty: Novice level

Preparation Time: 5 minutes

Cooking Time: 3 minutes

Serving: 2

Size/ Portion: 1 fillet

Ingredients:

Chutney:

- ¼ cup fresh dill
- ¼ cup extra virgin olive oil
- Juice from ½ lemon
- Sea salt, to taste

Fish:

- 2 cups water
- 2 salmon fillets

- Juice from ½ lemon
- ¼ teaspoon paprika
- Salt and freshly ground pepper to taste

Direction:

1. Pulse all the chutney ingredients in a food processor until creamy. Set aside.
2. Add the water and steamer basket to the Instant Pot. Place salmon fillets, skin-side down, on the steamer basket. Drizzle the lemon juice over salmon and sprinkle with the paprika.
3. Secure the lid. Select the Manual mode and set the cooking time for 3 minutes at High Pressure.
4. Once cooking is complete, do a quick pressure release. Carefully open the lid.
5. Season the fillets with pepper and salt to taste. Serve topped with the dill chutney.

Nutrition

636 calories

41g fat

65g protein

45g Carbohydrates

7. Garlic-Butter Parmesan Salmon and Asparagus

Difficulty: Novice level

Preparation Time: 10 minutes

Cooking Time: 15 minutes

Serving: 2

Size/ Portion: 1 fillet

Ingredients:

- 2 (6-ounce / 170-g) salmon fillets, skin on and patted dry
- Pink Himalayan salt
- Freshly ground black pepper, to taste
- 1 pound (454 g) fresh asparagus, ends snapped off
- 3 tablespoons almond butter

- 2 garlic cloves, minced
- ¼ cup grated Parmesan cheese

Direction:

1. Prep oven to 400°F (205°C). Line a baking sheet with aluminum foil.
2. Season both sides of the salmon fillets.
3. Situate salmon in the middle of the baking sheet and arrange the asparagus around the salmon.
4. Heat the almond butter in a small saucepan over medium heat.
5. Cook minced garlic
6. Drizzle the garlic-butter sauce over the salmon and asparagus and scatter the Parmesan cheese on top.
7. Bake in the preheated oven for about 12 minutes. You can switch the oven to broil at the end of cooking time for about 3 minutes to get a nice char on the asparagus.
8. Let cool for 5 minutes before serving.

Nutrition:

435 calories

26g fat

42g protein

68g Carbohydrates

8. Lemon Rosemary Roasted Branzino

Difficulty: Novice level

Preparation Time: 15 minutes

Cooking Time: 30 minutes

Serving: 2

Size/ Portion: 1 fillet

Ingredients:

- 4 tablespoons extra-virgin olive oil, divided
- 2 (8-ounce) Branzino fillets
- 1 garlic clove, minced

- 1 bunch scallions
- 10 to 12 small cherry tomatoes, halved
- 1 large carrot, cut into ¼-inch rounds
- ½ cup dry white wine
- 2 tablespoons paprika
- 2 teaspoons kosher salt
- ½ tablespoon ground chili pepper
- 2 rosemary sprigs or 1 tablespoon dried rosemary
- 1 small lemon, thinly sliced
- ½ cup sliced pitted kalamata olives

Direction:

1. Heat a large ovenproof skillet over high heat until hot, about 2 minutes. Add 1 tablespoon of olive oil and heat
2. Add the Branzino fillets, skin-side up, and sear for 2 minutes. Flip the fillets and cook. Set aside.
3. Swirl 2 tablespoons of olive oil around the skillet to coat evenly.
4. Add the garlic, scallions, tomatoes, and carrot, and sauté for 5 minutes
5. Add the wine, stirring until all ingredients are well combined. Carefully place the fish over the sauce.
6. Preheat the oven to 450°F (235°C).
7. Brush the fillets with the remaining 1 tablespoon of olive oil and season with paprika, salt, and chili pepper. Top each fillet with a rosemary sprig and lemon slices. Scatter the olives over fish and around the skillet.
8. Roast for about 10 minutes until the lemon slices are browned. Serve hot.

Nutrition:

724 calories

43g fat

57g protein

24g Carbohydrates

9. Grilled Lemon Pesto Salmon

Difficulty: Novice level

Preparation Time: 5 minutes

Cooking Time: 10 minutes

Serving: 2

Size/ Portion: 5 ounces

Ingredients:

- 10 ounces (283 g) salmon fillet
- 2 tablespoons prepared pesto sauce
- 1 large fresh lemon, sliced
- Cooking spray

Direction:

1. Preheat the grill to medium-high heat. Spray the grill grates with cooking spray.
2. Season the salmon well. Spread the pesto sauce on top.
3. Make a bed of fresh lemon slices about the same size as the salmon fillet on the hot grill, and place the salmon on top of the lemon slices. Put any additional lemon slices on top of the salmon.
4. Grill the salmon for 10 minutes.
5. Serve hot.

Nutrition:

316 calories

21g fat

29g protein

26g Carbohydrates

10. Steamed Trout with Lemon Herb Crust

Difficulty: Novice level

Preparation Time: 10 minutes

Cooking Time: 15 minutes

Serving: 2

Size/ Portion: 1 piece

Ingredients:

- 3 tablespoons olive oil

- 3 garlic cloves, chopped
- 2 tablespoons fresh lemon juice
- 1 tablespoon chopped fresh mint
- 1 tablespoon chopped fresh parsley
- ¼ teaspoon dried ground thyme
- 1 teaspoon sea salt
- 1 pound (454 g) fresh trout (2 pieces)
- 2 cups fish stock

Direction:

1. Blend olive oil, garlic, lemon juice, mint, parsley, thyme, and salt. Brush the marinade onto the fish.
2. Insert a trivet in the Instant Pot. Fill in the fish stock and place the fish on the trivet.
3. Secure the lid. Select the Steam mode and set the cooking time for 15 minutes at High Pressure.
4. Once cooking is complete, do a quick pressure release. Carefully open the lid. Serve warm.

Nutrition:

477 calories

30g fat

52g protein

27g Carbohydrates

11. Roasted Trout Stuffed with Veggies

Difficulty: Novice level

Preparation Time: 10 minutes

Cooking Time: 25 minutes

Serving: 2

Size/ Portion: 8 ounces

Ingredient:

- 2 (8-ounce) whole trout fillets
- 1 tablespoon extra-virgin olive oil
- ¼ teaspoon salt

- 1/8 teaspoon black pepper
- 1 small onion, thinly sliced
- ½ red bell pepper
- 1 poblano pepper
- 2 or 3 shiitake mushrooms, sliced
- 1 lemon, sliced

Direction:

1. Set oven to 425°F (220°C). Coat baking sheet with nonstick cooking spray.
2. Rub both trout fillets, inside and out, with the olive oil. Season with salt and pepper.
3. Mix together the onion, bell pepper, poblano pepper, and mushrooms in a large bowl. Stuff half of this mix into the cavity of each fillet. Top the mixture with 2 or 3 lemon slices inside each fillet.
4. Place the fish on the prepared baking sheet side by side. Roast in the preheated oven for 25 minutes
5. Pullout from the oven and serve on a plate.

Nutrition:

453 calories 22g fat

49g protein 35g Carbohydrates

12. Lemony Trout with Caramelized Shallots

Difficulty: Novice level

Preparation Time: 10 minutes

Cooking Time: 20 minutes

Serving: 2

Size/ Portion: 4 ounces

Ingredients:

Shallots:

- 1 teaspoon almond butter
- 2 shallots, thinly sliced
- Dash salt

Trout:

- 1 tablespoon almond butter
- 2 (4-ounce / 113-g) trout fillets
- 3 tablespoons capers
- ¼ cup freshly squeezed lemon juice
- ¼ teaspoon salt
- Dash freshly ground black pepper
- 1 lemon, thinly sliced

Direction:

For Shallots

1. Situate skillet over medium heat, cook the butter, shallots, and salt for 20 minutes, stirring every 5 minutes.

For Trout

2. Meanwhile, in another large skillet over medium heat, heat 1 teaspoon of almond butter.

3. Add the trout fillets and cook each side for 3 minutes, or until flaky. Transfer to a plate and set aside.

4. In the skillet used for the trout, stir in the capers, lemon juice, salt, and pepper, then bring to a simmer. Whisk in the remaining 1 tablespoon of almond butter. Spoon the sauce over the fish.

5. Garnish the fish with the lemon slices and caramelized shallots before serving.

Nutrition: 344 calories 18g fat 21g protein

37g Carbohydrates

13.   Easy Tomato Tuna Melts

Difficulty: Novice level

Preparation Time: 5 minutes

Cooking Time: 4 minutes

Serving: 2

Size/ Portion: 2.5 ounces

Ingredients:

- 1 (5-oz) can chunk light tuna packed in water

- 2 tablespoons plain Greek yogurt
- 2 tablespoons finely chopped celery
- 1 tablespoon finely chopped red onion
- 2 teaspoons freshly squeezed lemon juice
- 1 large tomato, cut into ¾-inch-thick rounds
- ½ cup shredded Cheddar cheese

Direction:

1. Preheat the broiler to High.

2. Stir together the tuna, yogurt, celery, red onion, lemon juice, and cayenne pepper in a medium bowl.

3. Place the tomato rounds on a baking sheet. Top each with some tuna salad and Cheddar cheese.

4. Broil for 3 to 4 minutes until the cheese is melted and bubbly. Cool for 5 minutes before serving.

Nutrition:

244 calories

10g fat

30g protein

26g Carbohydrates

14.   Mackerel and Green Bean Salad

Preparation Time: 10 minutes

Cooking Time: 10 minutes

Serving: 2

Size/ Portion: 2 cups

Ingredients:

- 2 cups green beans
- 1 tablespoon avocado oil
- 2 mackerel fillets
- 4 cups mixed salad greens
- 2 hard-boiled eggs, sliced
- 1 avocado, sliced
- 2 tablespoons lemon juice

- 2 tablespoons olive oil
- 1 teaspoon Dijon mustard
- Salt and black pepper, to taste

Direction:

1. Cook the green beans in pot of boiling water for about 3 minutes. Drain and set aside.
2. Melt the avocado oil in a pan over medium heat. Add the mackerel fillets and cook each side for 4 minutes.
3. Divide the greens between two salad bowls. Top with the mackerel, sliced egg, and avocado slices.
4. Scourge lemon juice, olive oil, mustard, salt, and pepper, and drizzle over the salad. Add the cooked green beans and toss to combine, then serve.

Nutrition:

737 calories

57g fat

34g protein

45g Carbohydrates

15. Hazelnut Crusted Sea Bass

Difficulty: Novice level

Preparation Time: 10 minutes

Cooking Time: 15 minutes

Serving: 2

Size/ Portion: 1 fillet

Ingredients:

- 2 tablespoons almond butter
- 2 sea bass fillets
- 1/3 cup roasted hazelnuts
- A pinch of cayenne pepper

Direction

1. Ready oven to 425°F (220°C). Line a baking dish with waxed paper.
2. Brush the almond butter over the fillets.

3. Pulse the hazelnuts and cayenne in a food processor. Coat the sea bass with the hazelnut mixture, then transfer to the baking dish.
4. Bake in the preheated oven for about 15 minutes. Cool for 5 minutes before serving.

Nutrition:

468 calories

31g fat

40g protein

38g Carbohydrates

16. Shrimp and Pea Paella

Difficulty: Novice level

Preparation Time: 20 minutes

Cooking Time: 60 minutes

Serving: 2

Size/ Portion: 4 ounces

Ingredients:

- 2 tablespoons olive oil
- 1 garlic clove, minced
- ½ large onion, minced
- 1 cup diced tomato
- ½ cup short-grain rice
- ½ teaspoon sweet paprika
- ½ cup dry white wine
- 1¼ cups low-sodium chicken stock
- 8 ounces (227 g) large raw shrimp
- 1 cup frozen peas
- ¼ cup jarred roasted red peppers

Direction

1. Heat the olive oil in a large skillet over medium-high heat.
2. Add the garlic and onion and sauté for 3 minutes, or until the onion is softened.
3. Add the tomato, rice, and paprika and stir for 3 minutes to toast the rice.

4. Add the wine and chicken stock and stir to combine. Bring the mixture to a boil.

5. Cover and set heat to medium-low, and simmer for 45 minutes

6. Add the shrimp, peas, and roasted red peppers. Cover and cook for an additional 5 minutes. Season with salt to taste and serve.

Nutrition:

646 calories

27g fat

42g protein

41g Carbohydrates

17. Garlic Shrimp with Arugula Pesto

Difficulty: Novice level

Preparation Time: 20 minutes

Cooking Time: 5 minutes

Serving: 2

Size/ Portion: 2 ounces

Ingredients:

- 3 cups lightly packed arugula
- ½ cup lightly packed basil leaves
- ¼ cup walnuts
- 3 tablespoons olive oil
- 3 medium garlic cloves
- 2 tablespoons grated Parmesan cheese
- 1 tablespoon freshly squeezed lemon juice
- 1 (10-ounce) package zucchini noodles
- 8 ounces (227 g) cooked, shelled shrimp
- 2 Roma tomatoes, diced

Direction

1. Process the arugula, basil, walnuts, olive oil, garlic, Parmesan cheese, and lemon juice in a food processor until smooth,

scraping down the sides as needed. Season

2. Heat a skillet over medium heat. Add the pesto, zucchini noodles, and cooked shrimp. Toss to combine the sauce over the noodles and shrimp, and cook until heated through.

3. Season well. Serve topped with the diced tomatoes.

Nutrition:

435 calories

30.2g fat

33g protein

38g Carbohydrates

18. Baked Oysters with Vegetables

Difficulty: Novice level

Preparation Time: 30 minutes

Cooking Time: 17 minutes

Serving: 2

Size/ Portion: 2 cups

Ingredients:

- 2 cups coarse salt, for holding the oysters
- 1 dozen fresh oysters, scrubbed
- 1 tablespoon almond butter
- ¼ cup finely chopped scallions
- ½ cup finely chopped artichoke hearts
- ¼ cup finely chopped red bell pepper
- 1 garlic clove, minced
- 1 tablespoon finely chopped fresh parsley
- Zest and juice of ½ lemon

Direction:

1. Pour the salt into a baking dish and spread to fill the bottom of the dish evenly.

2. Using a shucking knife, insert the blade at the joint of the shell, where it hinges open and shut. Firmly apply pressure to

pop the blade in, and work the knife around the shell to open. Discard the empty half of the shell. Using the knife, gently loosen the oyster, and remove any shell particles. Sprinkle salt in the oysters

3. Set oven to 425°F (220°C).

4. Heat the almond butter in a large skillet over medium heat. Add the scallions, artichoke hearts, and bell pepper, and cook for 5 to 7 minutes. Cook garlic

5. Takeout from the heat and stir in the parsley, lemon zest and juice, and season to taste with salt and pepper.

6. Divide the vegetable mixture evenly among the oysters. Bake in the preheated oven for 10 to 12 minutes.

Nutrition:

135 calories

7g fat

6g protein

7g Carbohydrates

19. Grilled Whole Sea Bass

Difficulty: Intermediate level

Preparation Time: 5 minutes

Cooking Time: 15 minutes

Serving: 2

Size/ portion: ½ lb.

Ingredients:

- 1 (1-pound) whole lavraki
- ¼ cup extra-virgin olive oil
- 1 bunch fresh thyme
- ¼ cup chopped fresh parsley
- 2 teaspoons minced garlic
- 1 small lemon, cut into ¼-inch rounds

Direction:

1. Preheat a grill to high heat.

2. Rub the olive oil all over the fish's surface and in its middle cavity.

3. Season liberally with salt and pepper.

4. Stuff the inner cavity with the thyme, parsley, garlic, and lemon slices.

5. Set the lavraki on the grill (see Cooking tip). Cook for 6 minutes per side.

6. Remove the head, backbone, and tail. Carve 2 fillets from each side for serving.

Nutrition:

480 Calories

34g Fat

43g Protein

28g Carbohydrates

20. Pan-Cooked Fish with Tomatoes

Difficulty: Intermediate level

Preparation Time: 20 minutes

Cooking Time: 45 minutes

Serving: 8

Size/ Portion: 3 ounces

Ingredients:

- 1½ cups extra-virgin olive oil
- 1½ cups tomato juice
- 2 (12-ounce) cans organic tomato paste
- 2 teaspoons sea salt
- 2 teaspoons cane sugar
- 1 teaspoon black pepper
- 1 teaspoon dried Greek oregano
- 3 pounds fresh white fish fillets
- 2 large sweet onions
- 1 cup white wine
- 1½ cups bread crumbs
- 4 garlic cloves
- ½ cup fresh parsley
- 4 large, firm tomatoes

Direction

1. Preheat the oven to 325°F.

2. Blend olive oil, tomato juice, tomato paste, salt, sugar, pepper, and oregano. Rub small amount of the mixture onto the bottom of 9-by-13-inch roasting pan.

3. Lay the fresh fish fillets side by side on top of the tomato mixture.

4. Cover with the onion slices, overlapping them.

5. Sprinkle the wine evenly over each piece of fish.

6. Pour half of the tomato and olive oil mixture over the fish.

7. Blend bread crumbs, garlic, and parsley. Spread over the fish.

8. Lay the tomato slices, overlapping them, over the fish. Drizzle remaining tomato mixture over the top.

9. Bake for 40 to 45 minutes.

Nutrition:

908 Calories 55g Fat

51g Protein 68g Carbohydrates

21. Fish Steamed in Parchment with Veggies

Difficulty: Intermediate level

Preparation Time: 25 minutes

Cooking Time: 20 minutes

Serving: 4

Size/ portion: 2 ounces

Ingredients:

- Juice of 2 lemons
- 4 tablespoons extra-virgin olive oil
- 2 teaspoons sea salt
- 1 teaspoon freshly ground black pepper
- 4 (6- to 8-ounce) fish fillets
- ½ pound tomatoes, chopped
- ½ cup chopped scallion

- ¼ cup chopped Kalamata olives
- 1 tablespoon capers, drained
- ¼ cup white wine vinegar
- 2 garlic cloves, minced
- 1 fennel bulb

Direction

1. Preheat the oven to 375°F.

2. Scourge lemon juice, 2 tablespoons of olive oil, salt, and pepper.

3. Add the fish and marinate in the refrigerator for 10 minutes.

4. In a medium bowl, combine the tomatoes, scallion, olives, capers, vinegar, remaining 2 tablespoons of olive oil, and garlic.

5. Fold 4 (12-by-16-inch) pieces of parchment paper in half and cut out a half heart shape, keeping as much of the parchment as possible. Unfold the hearts and place ¼ of the fennel close to the center crease to make a bed for the fish. Top with 1 fish fillet and ¼ of the tomato mixture.

6. Fold the parchment back over the fish and, starting at the bottom end, start folding the edges, overlapping to seal the packet. Bake for 20 minutes.

Nutrition:

277 Calories 16g Fat

27g Protein 17g Carbohydrates

22. Swordfish Souvlaki

Difficulty: Intermediate level

Preparation Time: 25 minutes

Cooking Time: 10 minutes

Serving: 4

Size/ portion: ½ lb.

Ingredients:

- ½ cup freshly squeezed lemon juice
- ½ cup extra-virgin olive oil

- 1 teaspoon kosher salt
- 1 teaspoon freshly ground black pepper
- 1 teaspoon dried Greek oregano
- 2 pounds swordfish steaks
- 8 ounces cherry tomatoes
- 1 red onion, quartered

Direction:

1. Scourge lemon juice, olive oil, salt, pepper, and oregano.

2. Add the fish and marinate in the refrigerator for 10 to 15 minutes.

3. Heat a grill to medium-high heat.

4. Skewer the swordfish, tomatoes, and red onion, alternating 1 to 2 pieces of fish for each tomato and onion quarter. Grill the kebabs for 10 minutes.

5. Alternatively, broil the skewers carefully for 3 to 5 minutes per side, checking frequently.

6. Serve with a squeeze of lemon and Avocado Skordalia / Avocado Garlic Spread.

Nutrition:

493 Calories

34g Fat

42g Protein

45g Carbohydrates

23. Stuffed Monkfish

Difficulty: Intermediate level

Preparation Time: 20 minutes

Cooking Time: 8 minutes

Serving: 4

Size/ portion: 6 ounces

Ingredients:

- 4 (6-ounce) fresh white fish fillets
- 6 tablespoons extra-virgin olive oil, divided

- ½ teaspoon sea salt
- ½ teaspoon freshly ground black pepper
- ¼ cup feta cheese
- ¼ cup minced green olives
- ¼ cup minced orange pulp
- 1 tablespoon orange zest
- ½ teaspoon dried dill
- ¼ cup chopped fresh Greek basil

Direction:

1. Blend fish with 2 tablespoons of olive oil, salt, and pepper.

2. In another bowl, mix together the feta, olives, and orange pulp. Spoon the mixture onto the fish fillets and spread it to coat them. Roll the fillets, inserting 2 toothpicks through to the other side to hold them together.

3. In heavy-bottomed skillet over medium-high heat, heat the remaining olive oil for about 15 seconds.

4. Add the rolled fillets and cook for 6 to 8 minutes, depending on their thickness, rolling onto each side as they cook.

5. Top each piece with the orange zest, dill, and basil, equally divided.

Nutrition:

365 Calories25g Fat

29g Protein

32g Carbohydrates

24. Shrimp Santorini

Difficulty: Intermediate level

Preparation Time: 20 minutes

Cooking Time: 30 minutes

Serving: 4

Size/ Portion: ¼ lb.

Ingredients:

- 1-pound shrimp
- 5 tablespoons extra-virgin olive oil

- 2 teaspoons kosher salt
- 2 teaspoons freshly ground black pepper
- 1 onion, chopped
- 4 garlic cloves, minced
- 2 pounds tomatoes, chopped or grated
- ½ teaspoon red pepper flakes
- ½ teaspoon dried Greek oregano
- 6 ounces feta cheese
- 3 tablespoons chopped fresh parsley

Direction:

1. Preheat the oven to 400°F.

2. Throw shrimp with 1 tablespoon of olive oil and the salt, and season with black pepper.

3. Using medium oven-safe skillet over medium heat, cook 4 tablespoons of olive oil.

4. Add the onion and season with salt. Cook for 3 to 5 minutes.

5. Add the garlic and black pepper. Cook for 4 minutes.

6. Cook tomatoes, red pepper flakes, and oregano for 10 minutes.

7. Arrange the shrimp and olives (if using) over the tomato mixture in one layer.

8. Crumble the feta over the surface.

9. Bake for 10 to 12 minutes.

10. Remove from the oven and garnish with parsley.

Nutrition:

458 Calories

29g Fat

35g Protein

32g Carbohydrates

25. Greek-Style Shrimp Cocktail

Difficulty: Intermediate level

Preparation Time: 15 minutes

Cooking Time: 5 minutes

Serving: 4

Size/ Portion: ¼ lb.

Ingredients:

- 1 pound (20- to 30-count) wild shrimp
- 1 egg
- 1 tablespoon Greek oregano or dill
- 2 teaspoons minced Kalamata olives
- 1 garlic clove, minced
- 1 teaspoon mustard
- ½ cup walnut oil
- ¼ teaspoon sea salt
- ¼ teaspoon freshly ground black pepper

Direction:

1. Boil 8 cups of water in pot over high heat.

2. Add the shrimp and boil for 2 to 3 minutes, until pink. Drain and cool.

3. In a food processor, combine the egg, oregano, olives, garlic, and mustard. Blend to combine.

4. With the processor running on low speed, very gradually add the walnut oil through the feed tube on your food processor.

5. When it has thickened to a mayonnaise-like texture, blend in the salt and pepper. Serve.

Nutrition:

257 Calories

13g Fat

31g Protein

24g Carbohydrates

26. Fried Calamari

Difficulty: Intermediate level

Preparation Time: 20 minutes

Cooking Time: 2 minutes

Serving: 6

Size/ Portion: ¼ lb.

Ingredient:

- 2 eggs
- 1 cup organic cornmeal
- 1 teaspoon sea salt
- ½ teaspoon dried dill
- 1-pound calamari rings and tentacles
- ½ cup Kalamata olives, pitted
- 1 lemon, cut into wedges and seeded
- 2 cups extra-virgin olive oil

Direction:

1. Beat the eggs in a flat shallow dish with a fork.

2. In another flat shallow dish, mix the cornmeal, salt, and dill with a fork.

3. Prepare the calamari, olives, and lemon slices for frying by lightly coating each piece with egg and dredging through the seasoned cornmeal.

4. With a skillet over medium heat, heat the olive oil

5. Add the calamari, lemon, and olives to the pan. Fry for about 2 minutes

6. Remove the items with a slotted spoon and place on paper towel to drain any excess oil.

Nutrition:

374 Calories

19g Fat

23g Protein

26g Carbohydrates

27. Stuffed Squid

Difficulty: Intermediate level

Preparation Time: 20 minutes

Cooking Time: 45 minutes

Serving: 4

Size/ Portion: ¼ lb.

Ingredients:

For squid

- 1 tablespoon extra-virgin olive oil
- 1 onion, chopped
- 1 teaspoon sea salt
- 1 teaspoon freshly ground black pepper
- 3 garlic cloves, minced
- 1-pound small squid
- ½ pound cherry tomatoes, halved
- ¼ cup basmati or long-grain rice, rinsed
- ¼ cup pine nuts, toasted
- ¼ cup fresh basil

For sauce

- ¼ cup extra-virgin olive oil
- 1 onion, chopped
- 1 teaspoon sea salt
- 1 teaspoon black pepper
- 2 garlic cloves, chopped
- ¼ cup dry white wine
- 1 (28-ounce) can diced tomatoes
- ¼ cup fresh basil, cut into chiffonade
- Juice of 1 lemon
- Lemon slices, for serving

Direction:

For squid

1. Situate pot over medium-high heat, heat the olive oil.

2. Sauté onion, salt, and pepper for 5 minutes.

3. Add the garlic. Cook for 1 minute

4. If the squid came with tentacles, chop them up and put them in the pot now.

5. Add the cherry tomatoes, rice, and pine nuts. Cook for 3 minutes

6. Fold the fresh basil into the mixture.

7. Prick the squid bodies all over with a toothpick and snip off the very end of the cavity.

8. Stuff each squid with filling so it is ¼- to-½ full. The rice will expand when the squid cooks in the sauce, so make sure there's room.

For sauce and cook the squid

1. In the same pot in which you cooked the stuffing, heat the olive oil over medium-high heat. 2. Add the onion, salt, and pepper. Cook for 3 to 5 minutes

3. Add the garlic. Cook for about 1 minute. 4. Stir white wine to deglaze the pan 5. Stir in the tomatoes. Cook for 10 minutes. 6. Add the basil.

7. Add the stuffed squid in even layers to the pot. Cover the pot and simmer for 30 minutes. Check the squid by piercing it with a knife—if there is too much resistance, cook for 15 minutes more.

8. When the squid is cooked through, squeeze the lemon into the pot and serve with additional lemon slices.

Nutrition: 429 Calories 25g Fat

22g Protein 32g Carbohydrates

28.   Octopus with Figs and Peaches

Difficulty: Intermediate level

Preparation Time: 15 minutes,

Cooking Time: 10 minutes

Serving: 4

Size/ Portion: ¼ lb.

Ingredient:

- 1-pound octopus tentacles

- ¼ cup extra-virgin olive oil
- 1 teaspoon sea salt
- 1 teaspoon black pepper
- 1 teaspoon granulated garlic
- ½ teaspoon dried Greek oregano
- 1 cup fig balsamic vinegar
- 6 fresh figs, halved
- 2 large peaches, quartered
- ¼ cup chopped fresh parsley

Direction:

1. In a large bowl, thoroughly mix the octopus, olive oil, salt, pepper, garlic, and oregano to coat well. Marinate in the refrigerator for 2 hours. Bring to room temperature before cooking.

2. In an 8- to 10-inch heavy-bottomed deep skillet over medium-high heat, bring the fig balsamic vinegar to a boil. Reduce the heat to a rolling simmer. Stir with the flat side of a metal spatula so any thickened vinegar is mixed into the liquid instead of sticking to the pan. After about 4 minutes, when the vinegar is foamy on top, add the octopus and stir quickly, cooking for only 2 to 3 minutes

3. Add the figs and peaches to the vinegar remaining in the skillet. Cook for about 1 minute, stirring them into the caramelized vinegar just until coated and soft. Transfer to the serving bowl and gently stir to combine.

4. Top with the parsley.

Nutrition:

304 Calories

14g Fat

21g Protein

18g Carbohydrates

29. Octopus with Potatoes

Difficulty: Professional level

Preparation Time: 10 minutes

Cooking Time: 35 minutes

Serving: 4

Size/ Portion: ½ lb.

Ingredients:

- 2 pounds octopus, cleaned
- 1-pound baby potatoes
- 1 fennel bulb, quartered
- 1 bay leaf
- 10 peppercorns
- Juice of 2 lemons
- ¼ cup extra-virgin olive oil
- 1 teaspoon kosher salt
- 1 teaspoon freshly ground black pepper
- 3 garlic cloves
- 1 cup chopped scallions
- ¼ cup chopped fresh parsley

Direction

1. Place 8-quart pot over medium-high heat, mix octopus, potatoes, fennel, bay leaf, and peppercorns. Cover with water. Cover the pot, bring to a boil, reduce the heat to low, and simmer. Don't overcook the octopus or it will be rubbery.

2. Preheat a grill to high heat.

3. Remove the octopus and cut it into 2- to 3-inch pieces and place them on the grill for 1 to 2 minutes per side.

4. In a medium bowl, whisk the lemon juice, olive oil, salt, pepper, and garlic.

5. Remove the potatoes from the pot and add to the dressing, along with the scallions and parsley, and toss to combine.

6. Add the grilled octopus to the bowl and toss with the rest of the ingredients. Turn out onto a platter and serve.

Nutrition:

392 Calories 15g Fat

43g Protein 11g Carbohydrates

30. Feta Crab Cakes

Difficulty: Professional level

Preparation Time: 30 minutes

Cooking Time: 15 minutes

Serving: 4

Size/ Portion: ¼ lb.

Ingredients:

- 1-pound crabmeat
- ½ cup minced scallion
- 1/3 cup bread crumbs
- ¼ cup feta cheese
- 2 eggs
- 2 garlic cloves
- 1 small Anaheim or pasilla chili
- 1 medium firm tomato
- 2 tablespoons minced fresh fennel
- 2 tablespoons minced fresh parsley
- ½ teaspoon dried dill
- ½ teaspoon dried Greek oregano
- ½ teaspoon sea salt
- ½ teaspoon freshly ground black pepper
- ¼ teaspoon ground nutmeg
- 3 tablespoons extra-virgin olive oil

Direction:

1. Blend crabmeat, scallion, bread crumbs, feta, eggs, garlic, chili, tomato, fennel, parsley, dill, oregano, salt, pepper, and nutmeg. Mix thoroughly. Split mixture into 8 equal portions and form each into a 2½-inch patty about ½ inch thick, creating a definitive edge for easier flipping when cooking.

2. Situate skillet over medium-high heat, heat the olive oil. Place the crab cakes in the heated pan and brown for 7 to 8 minutes per side.

Nutrition: 315 Calories 16g Fat

15g Protein 24g Carbohydrates

31. Steamed Mussels with White Wine and Fennel

Difficulty: Professional level

Preparation Time: 20 minutes

Cooking Time: 30 minutes

Serving: 4

Size/ Portion: 1 lb.

Ingredients:

- ¼ cup extra-virgin olive oil
- 1 onion, chopped
- 1 teaspoon sea salt
- 4 garlic cloves, minced
- 1 teaspoon red pepper flakes
- 1 fennel bulb
- 1 cup dry white wine
- 4 pounds mussels
- Juice of 2 lemons

Direction:

1. Position 8-quart pot over medium-high heat, heat the olive oil.

2. Add the onion and salt. Cook for 5 minutes, until translucent.

3. Add garlic and red pepper flakes. Cook for 1 minute.

4. Stir in the chopped fennel. Cook for 3 minutes.

5. Stir in the wine and simmer for about 7 minutes.

6. Carefully pour the mussels into the pot. Reduce the heat to medium, give everything a good stir, cover the pot, and cook for 5 to 7 minutes.

7. Remove the opened mussels and divide them among 4 bowls. Re-cover the pot and cook any unopened mussels for 3 minutes more. Divide any additional opened mussels among the bowls. Discard any unopened mussels. Evenly distribute the broth into the bowls. Garnish with the fennel leaves.

Nutrition: 578 Calories 23g Fat

55g Protein 35g Carbohydrates

32. Seafood Rice

Difficulty: Professional level

Preparation Time: 10 minutes

Cooking Time: 40 minutes

Serving: 6

Size/ Portion: ¼ lb.

Ingredients:

- 1 tablespoon extra-virgin olive oil
- 1½ pounds seafood
- 1 onion, chopped
- 1 teaspoon sea salt
- 4 garlic cloves, minced
- 1 cup chopped celery
- 2 medium tomatoes
- ½ cup dry white wine
- 2 cups arborio rice
- ¼ cup chopped fresh parsley
- ¼ cup chopped fresh dill
- 4¼ cups chicken broth

Direction:

1. Put skillet over medium-high heat, heat 1 tablespoon of olive oil.

2. Add the squid and cook for about 2 minutes. Remove the squid and set aside.

3. Add the remaining 1 teaspoon of olive oil to the skillet to heat.

4. Add the onion and salt. Cook for 5 minutes.

5. Cook garlic.

6. Add the celery and tomatoes. Cook for 3 minutes.

7. Pour in the wine and cook for about 3 minutes, stirring frequently.

8. Stir in the rice, parsley, dill, and 4 cups of broth. Cover the skillet and simmer for 15 minutes.

9. Top the rice mixture with the shrimp and mussels, cover the skillet, and simmer for 5 minutes more, until the shrimp are just cooked.

10. Return the squid to the skillet. Discard any unopened mussels. Side with the lemon wedges

Nutrition: 246 Calories 5g Fat

28g Protein 24g Carbohydrates

33. Mixed Seafood with Wine and Capers

Difficulty: Professional level

Preparation Time: 25 minutes

Cooking Time: 10 minutes

Serving: 4

Size/ Portion: ¼ lb.

Ingredients:

- 1 (1-pound) bag frozen mixed seafood
- ½ cup white wine
- ¼ cup extra-virgin olive oil
- ½ teaspoon sea salt
- ½ teaspoon freshly ground black pepper
- ½ cup capers, drained
- ¼ cup chopped fresh parsley

Direction:

1. Thaw the frozen seafood by rinsing in a colander under cold running water for several minutes, turning so that it will thaw evenly. Put aside for 5 minutes, and squeeze out excess water completely.

2. In a small bowl, whisk the white wine, olive oil, salt, and pepper.

3. In a 10-inch skillet over medium-high heat, bring the white wine mixture to a simmer.

4. Add the seafood and stir in the capers. Cook for 5 minutes.

5. Sprinkle with the parsley and serve.

Nutrition: 235 Calories 14g Fat

17g Protein 18g Carbohydrates

Lunch and Dinner (Vegetable Recipes)

1. Rice with Vermicelli

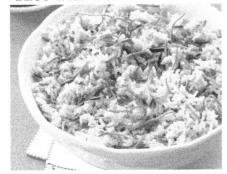

Difficulty: Novice level

Preparation Time: 5 minutes

Cooking Time: 45 minutes

Serving: 6

Size/ portion: 1 cup

Ingredients

- 2 cups short-grain rice
- 3½ cups water
- ¼ cup olive oil
- 1 cup broken vermicelli pasta
- Salt

Direction

1. Rinse the rice under cold water until the water runs clean. Place the rice in a bowl, cover with water, and let soak for 10 minutes. Drain and set aside.

2. In a medium pot over medium heat, heat the olive oil.

3. Stir in the vermicelli and cook for 2 to 3 minutes, stirring continuously, until golden.

4. Add the rice and cook for 1 minute, stirring, so the rice is well coated in the oil.

5. Add the water and a pinch of salt and bring the liquid to a boil. Reduce the heat to low, cover the pot, and simmer for 20 minutes.

6. Remove from the heat and let rest, covered, for 10 minutes. Fluff with a fork and serve.

Nutrition:

346 calories

9g fat

7g protein

6g Carbohydrates

2. Fava Beans and Rice

Difficulty: Novice level

Preparation Time: 10 minutes

Cooking Time: 35 minutes

Serving: 4

Size/ portion: 1 cup

Ingredients:

- ¼ cup olive oil
- 4 cups fresh fava beans
- 4½ cups water
- 2 cups basmati rice
- 1/8 teaspoon salt
- 1/8 teaspoon black pepper

- 2 tablespoons pine nuts, toasted
- ½ cup chopped fresh garlic chives

Direction:

1. In a large saucepan over medium heat, heat the olive oil.

2. Add the fava beans and drizzle them with a bit of water. Cook for 10 minutes.

3. Gently stir in the rice. Add the water, salt, and pepper. Increase the heat and bring the mixture to a boil. Cover, reduce the heat to low, and simmer for 15 minutes.

4. Turn off the heat and let the mixture rest for 10 minutes before serving. Sprinkle with toasted pine nuts and chives.

Nutrition: 587 calories17g fat

17g protein. 14g Carbohydrates

3. Buttered Fava Beans

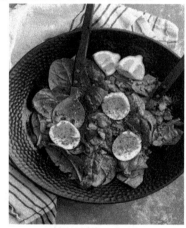

Difficulty: Novice level

Preparation Time: 30 minutes

Cooking Time: 15 minutes

Serving: 4

Size/ Portion: ½ cup

Ingredients

- ½ cup vegetable broth
- 4 pounds fava beans
- ¼ cup fresh tarragon
- 1 teaspoon chopped fresh thyme

- ¼ teaspoon black pepper
- 1/8 teaspoon salt
- 2 tablespoons butter
- 1 garlic clove, minced
- 2 tablespoons chopped fresh parsley

Direction:

1. In a shallow pan over medium heat, bring the vegetable broth to a boil.
2. Add the fava beans, 2 tablespoons of tarragon, the thyme, pepper, and salt. Cook for 10 minutes.
3. Stir in the butter, garlic, and remaining 2 tablespoons of tarragon. Cook for 2 to 3 minutes.
4. Sprinkle with the parsley.

Nutrition: 458 calories 9g fat

37g protein 27g Carbohydrates

4. Freekeh

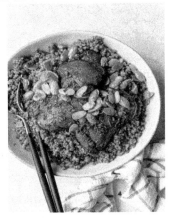

Difficulty: Novice level

Preparation Time: 10 minutes

Cooking Time: 40 minutes

Scrving: 4

Size/ portion: ½ cup

Ingredients:

- 4 tablespoons Ghee
- 1 onion, chopped
- 3½ cups vegetable broth

- 1 teaspoon ground allspice
- 2 cups freekeh
- 2 tablespoons pine nuts

Direction

1. In a heavy-bottomed saucepan over medium heat, melt the ghee.
2. Stir in the onion and cook for about 5 minutes, stirring constantly, until the onion is golden.
3. Pour in the vegetable broth, add the allspice, and bring to a boil.
4. Stir in the freekeh and return the mixture to a boil. Reduce the heat to low, cover the pan, and simmer for 30 minutes, stirring occasionally.
5. Spoon the freekeh into a serving dish and top with the toasted pine nuts.

Nutrition:

459 calories

18g fat

19g protein

14g Carbohydrates

5. Fried Rice Balls with Tomato Sauce

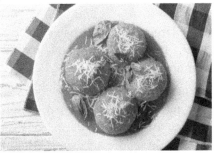

Difficulty: Novice level

Preparation Time: 15 minutes

Cooking Time: 20 minutes

Serving: 4

Size/ portion: 2 balls

Ingredients:

- 1 cup bread crumbs

- 2 cups cooked risotto
- 2 large eggs, divided
- ¼ cup freshly grated Parmesan cheese
- 8 fresh baby mozzarella balls
- 2 tablespoons water
- 1 cup corn oil
- 1 cup Basic Tomato Basil Sauce

Direction

1. Pour the bread crumbs into a small bowl and set aside.
2. In a medium bowl, stir together the risotto, 1 egg, and the Parmesan cheese until well combined.
3. Moisten your hands with a little water to prevent sticking and divide the risotto mixture into 8 pieces. Place them on a clean work surface and flatten each piece.
4. Place 1 mozzarella ball on each flattened rice disk. Close the rice around the mozzarella to form a ball. Repeat until you finish all the balls.
5. In the same medium, now-empty bowl, whisk the remaining egg and the water.
6. Dip each prepared risotto ball into the egg wash and roll it in the bread crumbs. Set aside.
7. In a large sauté pan or skillet over high heat, heat the corn oil for about 3 minutes.
8. Gently lower the risotto balls into the hot oil and fry for 5 to 8 minutes until golden brown. Stir them, as needed, to ensure the entire surface is fried. Using a slotted spoon, transfer the fried balls to paper towels to drain.
9. In a medium saucepan over medium heat, heat the tomato sauce for 5 minutes, stirring occasionally, and serve the warm sauce alongside the rice balls.

Nutrition: 255 calories 15g fat
11g protein 13g Carbohydrates

6.   Spanish-Style Rice

Difficulty: Novice level

Preparation Time: 10 minutes

Cooking Time: 35 minutes

Serving: 4

Size/ Portion: 2 cups

Ingredients:

- ¼ cup olive oil
- 1 small onion
- 1 red bell pepper
- 1½ cups white rice
- 1 teaspoon sweet paprika
- ½ teaspoon ground cumin
- ½ teaspoon ground coriander
- 1 garlic clove, minced
- 3 tablespoons tomato paste
- 3 cups vegetable broth
- 1/8 teaspoon salt

Direction:

1. In a large heavy-bottomed skillet over medium heat, heat the olive oil.
2. Stir in the onion and red bell pepper. Cook for 5 minutes or until softened.
3. Add the rice, paprika, cumin, and coriander and cook for 2 minutes, stirring often.
4. Add the garlic, tomato paste, vegetable broth, and salt. Stir to combine, taste, and season with more salt, as needed.
5. Increase the heat to bring the mixture to a boil. Reduce the heat to low, cover the skillet, and simmer for 20 minutes.
6. Let the rice rest, covered, for 5 minutes before serving.

Nutrition:

414 calories 14g fat

6g protein

8g Carbohydrates

7.   Zucchini with Rice and Tzatziki

Difficulty: Novice level

Preparation Time: 20 minutes

Cooking Time: 35 minutes

Serving: 4

Size/ Portion: 2 cups

Ingredients:

- ¼ cup olive oil
- 1 onion
- 3 zucchinis
- 1 cup vegetable broth
- ½ cup chopped fresh dill
- 1 cup short-grain rice
- 2 tablespoons pine nuts
- 1 cup Tzatziki Sauce, Plain Yogurt

Direction:

1. In a heavy-bottomed pot over medium heat, heat the olive oil.
2. Add the onion, turn the heat to medium-low, and sauté for 5 minutes.
3. Add the zucchini and cook for 2 minutes more.
4. Stir in the vegetable broth and dill and season with salt and pepper. Increase the heat to medium and bring the mixture to a boil.
5. Stir in the rice and let it boil. Set to very low heat, cover the pot, and cook for 15 minutes. Remove from the heat and let the rice rest, covered, for 10 minutes.
6. Spoon the rice onto a serving platter, sprinkle with the pine nuts, and serve with tzatziki sauce.

Nutrition:

414 calories

17g fat

11g protein

19g Carbohydrates

8.   Cannellini Beans with Rosemary and Garlic Aioli

Difficulty: Novice level

Preparation Time: 10 minutes

Cooking Time: 10 minutes

Serving: 4

Size/ Portion: ½ cup

Ingredients:

- 4 cups cooked cannellini beans
- 4 cups water
- ½ teaspoon salt
- 3 tablespoons olive oil
- 2 tablespoons chopped fresh rosemary
- ½ cup Garlic Aioli
- ¼ teaspoon freshly ground black pepper

Direction:

1. In a medium saucepan over medium heat, combine the cannellini beans, water, and salt. Bring to a boil. Cook for 5 minutes. Drain.
2. In a skillet over medium heat, heat the olive oil.
3. Add the beans. Stir in the rosemary and aioli. Reduce the heat to medium-low and cook, stirring, just to heat through. Season with pepper and serve.

Nutrition: 545 calories 36g fat

15g protein 25g Carbohydrates

9.   Jeweled Rice

Difficulty: Novice level

Preparation Time: 15 minutes

Cooking Time: 30 minutes

Serving: 6

Size/ Portion: 2 cups

Ingredients:

- ½ cup olive oil, divided
- 1 onion, finely chopped

- 1 garlic clove, minced
- ½ teaspoon fresh ginger
- 4½ cups water
- 1 teaspoon salt
- 1 teaspoon ground turmeric
- 2 cups basmati rice
- 1 cup fresh sweet peas
- 2 carrots
- ½ cup dried cranberries
- Grated zest of 1 orange
- 1/8 teaspoon cayenne pepper
- ¼ cup slivered almonds

Direction:

1. In a large heavy-bottomed pot over medium heat, heat ¼ cup of olive oil.

2. Add the onion and cook for 4 minutes. Add the garlic and ginger and cook for 1 minute more.

3. Stir in the water, ¾ teaspoon of salt, and the turmeric. Bring the mixture to a boil. Mix in the rice and boil. Select heat to low, cover the pot, and cook for 15 minutes. Turn off the heat. Let the rice rest on the burner, covered, for 10 minutes.

4. Meanwhile, in a medium sauté pan or skillet over medium-low heat, heat the remaining ¼ cup of olive oil. Stir in the peas and carrots. Cook for 5 minutes.

5. Stir in the cranberries and orange zest. Season with the remaining ¼ teaspoon of salt and the cayenne. Cook for 1 to 2 minutes.

6. Spoon the rice onto a serving platter. Top with the peas and carrots and sprinkle with the toasted almonds.

Nutrition:

460 calories 19g fat

7g protein 10g Carbohydrates

10.   Asparagus Risotto

Difficulty: Novice level

Preparation Time: 15 minutes

Cooking Time: 30 minutes

Serving: 4

Size/ Portion: 2 cups

Ingredients:

- 5 cups vegetable broth
- 3 tablespoons unsalted butter
- 1 tablespoon olive oil
- 1 small onion, chopped
- 1½ cups Arborio rice
- 1-pound fresh asparagus
- ¼ cup freshly grated Parmesan cheese, plus more for serving

Direction:

1. In a saucepan over medium heat, bring the vegetable broth to a boil. Turn the heat to low and keep the broth at a steady simmer.

2. In a 4-quart heavy-bottomed saucepan over medium heat, melt 2 tablespoons of butter with the olive oil. Add the onion and cook for 2 to 3 minutes.

3. Add the rice and stir with a wooden spoon while cooking for 1 minute until the grains are well coated in the butter and oil.

4. Stir in ½ cup of warm broth. Cook, stirring often, for about 5 minutes until the broth is completely absorbed.

5. Add the asparagus stalks and another ½ cup of broth. Cook, stirring often, until the liquid is absorbed. Continue adding the broth, ½ cup at a time, and cooking until it is completely absorbed before adding the next ½ cup. Stir frequently to prevent sticking. After about 20 minutes, the rice should be cooked but still firm.

6. Add the asparagus tips, the remaining 1 tablespoon of butter, and the Parmesan cheese. Stir vigorously to combine.

7. Remove from the heat, top with additional Parmesan cheese, if desired, and serve immediately.

Nutrition:

434 calories

14g fat

10g protein

13g Carbohydrates

11. Vegetable Paella

Difficulty: Novice level

Preparation Time: 25 minutes

Cooking Time: 45 minutes

Serving: 6

Size/ Portion: 2 cups

Ingredients:

- ¼ cup olive oil
- 1 large sweet onion
- 1 large red bell pepper
- 1 large green bell pepper
- 3 garlic cloves
- 1 teaspoon smoked paprika
- 5 saffron threads
- 1 zucchini, cut into ½-inch cubes
- 4 large ripe tomatoes
- 1½ cups short-grain Spanish rice
- 3 cups vegetable broth, warmed

Direction:

1. Preheat the oven to 350°F.

2. In a paella pan or large oven-safe skillet over medium heat, heat the olive oil.

3. Add the onion and red and green bell peppers and cook for 10 minutes.

4. Stir in the garlic, paprika, saffron threads, zucchini, and tomatoes. Turn the heat to medium-low and cook for 10 minutes.

5. Stir in the rice and vegetable broth. Increase the heat to bring the paella to a boil. Reduce the heat to medium-low and cook for 15 minutes. Cover the pan with aluminum foil and put it in the oven.

6. Bake for 10 minutes or until the broth is absorbed.

Nutrition:

288 calories 10g fat

5g protein

15g Carbohydrates

12. Eggplant and Rice Casserole

Difficulty: Novice level

Preparation Time: 30 minutes

Cooking Time: 35 minutes

Serving: 4

Size/ Portion: 2 cups

Ingredients:

For sauce

- ½ cup olive oil
- 1 small onion
- 4 garlic cloves
- 6 ripe tomatoes
- 2 tablespoons tomato paste
- 1 teaspoon dried oregano
- ¼ teaspoon ground nutmeg
- ¼ teaspoon ground cumin

For casserole

- 4 (6-inch) Japanese eggplants
- 2 tablespoons olive oil
- 1 cup cooked rice
- 2 tablespoons pine nuts
- 1 cup water

Direction:

For sauce

1. In a heavy-bottomed saucepan over medium heat, heat the olive oil. Add the onion and cook for 5 minutes.

2. Stir in the garlic, tomatoes, tomato paste, oregano, nutmeg, and cumin. Bring to a boil. Cover, reduce heat to low, and simmer for 10 minutes. Remove and set aside.

For casserole

3. Preheat the broiler.

4. While the sauce simmers, drizzle the eggplant with the olive oil and place them on a baking sheet. Broil for about 5 minutes until golden. Remove and let cool.

5. Turn the oven to 375°F. Arrange the cooled eggplant, cut-side up, in a 9-by-13-inch baking dish. Gently scoop out some flesh to make room for the stuffing.

6. In a bowl, combine half the tomato sauce, the cooked rice, and pine nuts. Fill each eggplant half with the rice mixture.

7. In the same bowl, combine the remaining tomato sauce and water. Pour over the eggplant.

8. Bake, covered, for 20 minutes.

Nutrition:

453 calories 39g fat

6g protein 14g Carbohydrates

13.   Many Vegetable Couscous

Difficulty: Novice level

Preparation Time: 15 minutes

Cooking Time: 45 minutes

Serving: 8

Size/ Portion: 1 cup

Ingredients:

- ¼ cup olive oil
- 1 onion, chopped
- 4 garlic cloves, minced
- 2 jalapeño peppers
- ½ teaspoon ground cumin
- ½ teaspoon ground coriander
- 1 (28-ounce) can crushed tomatoes
- 2 tablespoons tomato paste
- 1/8 teaspoon salt
- 2 bay leaves
- 11 cups water, divided
- 4 carrots, peeled and cut into 2-inch pieces
- 2 zucchinis
- 1 acorn squash
- 1 (15-ounce) can chickpeas
- ¼ cup chopped Preserved Lemons (optional)
- 3 cups couscous

Direction:

1. In a large heavy-bottomed pot over medium heat, heat the olive oil. Stir in the onion and cook for 4 minutes. Stir in the garlic, jalapeños, cumin, and coriander. Cook for 1 minute.

2. Add the tomatoes, tomato paste, salt, bay leaves, and 8 cups of water. Bring the mixture to a boil.

3. Add the carrots, zucchini, and acorn squash and return to a boil. Reduce the heat slightly, cover, and cook for about 20 minutes until the vegetables are tender but not mushy. Remove 2 cups of the cooking liquid and set aside. Season as needed.

4. Add the chickpeas and preserved lemons (if using). Cook for 2 to 3 minutes, and turn off the heat.

5. In a medium pan, bring the remaining 3 cups of water to a boil over high heat.

Stir in the couscous, cover, and turn off the heat. Let the couscous rest for 10 minutes. Drizzle with 1 cup of reserved cooking liquid. Using a fork, fluff the couscous.

6. Mound it on a large platter. Drizzle it with the remaining cooking liquid. Remove the vegetables from the pot and arrange on top. Serve the remaining stew in a separate bowl.

Nutrition:

415 calories 7g fat

14g protein 17g Carbohydrates

14. Kushari

Difficulty: Novice level

Preparation Time: 25 minutes

Cooking Time: 80 minutes

Serving: 8

Size/ Portion: 1 cup

Ingredients:

For sauce

- 2 tablespoons olive oil
- 2 garlic cloves, minced
- 1 (16-ounce) can tomato sauce
- ¼ cup white vinegar
- ¼ cup Harissa, or store-bought
- 1/8 teaspoon salt

For rice

- 1 cup olive oil
- 2 onions, thinly sliced
- 2 cups dried brown lentils
- 4 quarts plus ½ cup water
- 2 cups short-grain rice
- 1 teaspoon salt
- 1-pound short elbow pasta
- 1 (15-ounce) can chickpeas

Direction:

For sauce

1. In a saucepan over medium heat, heat the olive oil.

2. Add the garlic and cook for 1 minute.

3. Stir in the tomato sauce, vinegar, harissa, and salt. Increase the heat to bring the sauce to a boil. Reduce the heat to low and cook for 20 minutes or until the sauce has thickened. Remove and set aside.

For rice

4. Line a plate with paper towels and set aside.

5. In a large pan over medium heat, heat the olive oil.

6. Add the onions and cook for 7 to 10 minutes, stirring often, until crisp and golden. Transfer the onions to the prepared plate and set aside. Reserve 2 tablespoons of the cooking oil. Reserve the pan.

7. In a large pot over high heat, combine the lentils and 4 cups of water. Bring to a boil and cook for 20 minutes. Drain, transfer to a bowl, and toss with the reserved 2 tablespoons of cooking oil. Set aside. Reserve the pot.

8. Place the pan you used to fry the onions over medium-high heat and add the rice, 4½ cups of water, and the salt to it. Bring to a boil. Reduce the heat to low, cover the pot, and cook for 20 minutes. Turn off the heat and let the rice rest for 10 minutes.6.

9. In the pot used to cook the lentils, bring the remaining 8 cups of water, salted, to a boil over high heat. Drop in the pasta and cook for 6 minutes or according to the package instructions. Drain and set aside.

10. To assemble: Spoon the rice onto a serving platter. Top it with the lentils, chickpeas, and pasta. Drizzle with the hot tomato sauce and sprinkle with the crispy fried onions.

Nutrition:

668 calories

13g fat

25g protein

21g Carbohydrates

15. Bulgur with Tomatoes and Chickpeas

Difficulty: Novice level

Preparation Time: 10 minutes

Cooking Time: 35 minutes

Serving: 6

Size/ Portion: 1 cup

Ingredients:

- ½ cup olive oil
- 1 onion, chopped
- 6 tomatoes
- 2 tablespoons tomato paste
- 2 cups water
- 1 tablespoon Harissa
- 1/8 teaspoon salt
- 2 cups coarse bulgur #3
- 1 (15-ounce) can chickpeas

Direction:

1. In a heavy-bottomed pot over medium heat, heat the olive oil.
2. Add the onion and sauté for 5 minutes.
3. Add the tomatoes with their juice and cook for 5 minutes.
4. Stir in the tomato paste, water, harissa, and salt. Bring to a boil.
5. Stir in the bulgur and chickpeas. Return the mixture to a boil. Reduce the heat to

low, cover the pot, and cook for 15 minutes. Let rest for 15 minutes before serving.

Nutrition:

413 calories

19g fat

11g protein

15g Carbohydrates

16. Portobello Caprese

Difficulty: Intermediate level

Preparation Time: 15 minutes

Cooking Time: 30 minutes

Serving: 2

Size/ Portion: 1 piece

Ingredient:

- 1 tablespoon olive oil
- 1 cup cherry tomatoes
- 4 large fresh basil leaves, thinly sliced, divided
- 3 medium garlic cloves, minced
- 2 large portobello mushrooms, stems removed
- 4 pieces mini Mozzarella balls
- 1 tablespoon Parmesan cheese, grated

Direction:

1. Prep oven to 350°F (180°C). Grease a baking pan with olive oil.
2. Drizzle 1 tablespoon olive oil in a nonstick skillet, and heat over medium-high heat.
3. Add the tomatoes to the skillet, and sprinkle salt and black pepper to season. Prick some holes on the tomatoes for juice during the cooking. Put the lid on and cook the tomatoes for 10 minutes or until tender.
4. Reserve 2 teaspoons of basil and add the remaining basil and garlic to the skillet.

Crush the tomatoes with a spatula, then cook for half a minute. Stir constantly during the cooking. Set aside.

5. Arrange the mushrooms in the baking pan, cap side down, and sprinkle with salt and black pepper to taste.

6. Spoon the tomato mixture and Mozzarella balls on the gill of the mushrooms, then scatter with Parmesan cheese to coat well.

7. Bake for 20 minutes

8. Remove the stuffed mushrooms from the oven and serve with basil on top.

Nutrition

285 calories

21.8g fat

14.3g protein

14.2g Carbohydrates

17. Mushroom and Cheese Stuffed Tomatoes

Difficulty: Intermediate level

Preparation Time: 15 minutes

Cooking Time: 20 minutes

Serving: 4

Size/ Portion: 1 piece

Ingredients:

- 4 large ripe tomatoes
- 1 tablespoon olive oil
- ½ pound (454 g) white or cremini mushrooms
- 1 tablespoon fresh basil, chopped
- ½ cup yellow onion, diced
- 1 tablespoon fresh oregano, chopped
- 2 garlic cloves, minced
- ½ teaspoon salt
- ¼ teaspoon freshly ground black pepper

- 1 cup part-skim Mozzarella cheese, shredded
- 1 tablespoon Parmesan cheese, grated

Direction:

1. Set oven to 375°F (190°C).

2. Chop a ½-inch slice off the top of each tomato. Scoop the pulp into a bowl and leave ½-inch tomato shells. Arrange the tomatoes on a baking sheet lined with aluminum foil.

3. Heat the olive oil in a nonstick skillet over medium heat.

4. Add the mushrooms, basil, onion, oregano, garlic, salt, and black pepper to the skillet and sauté for 5 minutes

5. Pour the mixture to the bowl of tomato pulp, then add the Mozzarella cheese and stir to combine well.

6. Spoon the mixture into each tomato shell, then top with a layer of Parmesan.

7. Bake for 15 minutes

8. Remove the stuffed tomatoes from the oven and serve warm.

Nutrition:

254 calories

14.7g fat

17.5g protein

18.6g Carbohydrates

18. Tabbouleh

Difficulty: Intermediate level

Preparation Time: 15 minutes

Cooking Time: 5 minutes

Serving: 6

Size/ Portion: 2 cups

Ingredients:

- 4 tablespoons olive oil
- 4 cups riced cauliflower
- 3 garlic cloves

- ½ large cucumber
- ½ cup Italian parsley
- Juice of 1 lemon
- 2 tablespoons red onion
- ½ cup mint leaves, chopped
- ½ cup pitted Kalamata olives
- 1 cup cherry tomatoes
- 2 cups baby arugula
- 2 medium avocados

Direction:

1. Warm 2 tablespoons olive oil in a nonstick skillet over medium-high heat.
2. Add the rice cauliflower, garlic, salt, and black pepper to the skillet and sauté for 3 minutes or until fragrant. Transfer them to a large bowl.
3. Add the cucumber, parsley, lemon juice, red onion, mint, olives, and remaining olive oil to the bowl. Toss to combine well. Reserve the bowl in the refrigerator for at least 30 minutes.
4. Remove the bowl from the refrigerator. Add the cherry tomatoes, arugula, and avocado to the bowl. Sprinkle with salt and black pepper, and toss to combine well. Serve chilled.

Nutrition:

198 calories 17.5g fat

4.2g protein 8.9g Carbohydrates

19. Spicy Broccoli Rabe and Artichoke Hearts

Difficulty: Intermediate level

Preparation Time: 5 minutes

Cooking Time: 15 minutes

Serving: 4

Size/ Portion: ½ lb.

Ingredient:

- 3 tablespoons olive oil, divided

- 2 pounds fresh broccoli rabe
- 3 garlic cloves, finely minced
- 1 teaspoon red pepper flakes
- 1 teaspoon salt, plus more to taste
- 13.5 ounces artichoke hearts
- 1 tablespoon water
- 2 tablespoons red wine vinegar

Direction:

1. Warm 2 tablespoons olive oil in a nonstick skillet over medium-high skillet.
2. Add the broccoli, garlic, red pepper flakes, and salt to the skillet and sauté for 5 minutes or until the broccoli is soft.
3. Add the artichoke hearts to the skillet and sauté for 2 more minutes or until tender.
4. Add water to the skillet and turn down the heat to low. Put the lid on and simmer for 5 minutes.
5. Meanwhile, combine the vinegar and 1 tablespoon of olive oil in a bowl.
6. Drizzle the simmered broccoli and artichokes with oiled vinegar, and sprinkle with salt and black pepper. Toss to combine well before serving.

Nutrition:

272 calories 21.5g fat

11.2g protein

12.3g Carbohydrates

20. Shakshuka

Difficulty: Intermediate level

Preparation Time: 10 minutes

Cooking Time: 25 minutes

Serving: 4

Size/ portion: 1 cup

Ingredient:

- 5 tablespoons olive oil, divided
- 1 red bell pepper, finely diced

- ½ small yellow onion, finely diced
- 14 ounces crushed tomatoes, with juices
- 6 ounces frozen spinach
- 1 teaspoon smoked paprika
- 2 garlic cloves
- 2 teaspoons red pepper flakes
- 1 tablespoon capers
- 1 tablespoon water
- 6 large eggs
- ¼ teaspoon freshly ground black pepper
- ¾ cup feta or goat cheese
- ¼ cup fresh flat-leaf parsley

Direction:

1. Prep oven to 300°F (150°C).
2. Cook 2 tablespoons olive oil in an oven-safe skillet over medium-high heat.
3. Cook bell pepper and onion to the skillet for 6 minutes.
4. Add the tomatoes and juices, spinach, paprika, garlic, red pepper flakes, capers, water, and 2 tablespoons olive oil to the skillet. Stir and boil.
5. Turn down the heat to low, then put the lid on and simmer for 5 minutes.
6. Crack the eggs over the sauce, and keep a little space between each egg, leave the egg intact and sprinkle with freshly ground black pepper.
7. Cook for another 8 minutes
8. Scatter the cheese over the eggs and sauce, and bake in the preheated oven for 5 minutes
9. Drizzle 1 tablespoon olive oil and spread the parsley on top before serving warm.

Nutrition:

335 calories 26.5g fat

16.8g protein

23.4g Carbohydrates

21.   Spanakopita

Difficulty: Intermediate level

Preparation Time: 15 minutes

Cooking Time: 50 minutes

Serving: 6

Size/ Portion: 1 cup

Ingredients:

- 6 tablespoons olive oil
- 1 small yellow onion
- 4 cups frozen chopped spinach
- 4 garlic cloves, minced
- ½ teaspoon salt
- ½ teaspoon freshly ground black pepper
- 4 large eggs, beaten
- 1 cup ricotta cheese
- ¾ cup feta cheese, crumbled
- ¼ cup pine nuts

Direction

1. Set oven to 375°F (190°C). Coat a baking dish with 2 tablespoons olive oil.
2. Heat 2 tablespoons olive oil in a nonstick skillet over medium-high heat.
3. Add the onion to the skillet and sauté for 6 minutes or until translucent and tender.
4. Add the spinach, garlic, salt, and black pepper to the skillet and sauté for 5 minutes more. Keep aside
5. Combine the beaten eggs and ricotta cheese in a separate bowl, then pour them in to the bowl of spinach mixture. Stir to mix well.
6. Pour the mixture into the baking dish, and tilt the dish so the mixture coats the bottom evenly.
7. Bake for 20 minutes. Remove the baking dish from the oven, and spread the feta cheese and pine nuts on top, then drizzle with remaining 2 tablespoons olive oil.

8. Return the baking dish to the oven and bake for another 15 minutes

9. Remove the dish from the oven. Allow the spanakopita to cool for a few minutes and slice to serve.

Nutrition:

340 calories

27.3g fat

18.2g protein

23.2g Carbohydrates

22. Tagine

Difficulty: Intermediate level

Preparation Time: 20 minutes

Cooking Time: 1 hour

Serving: 6

Size/ Portion: 1 cup

Ingredients:

- ½ cup olive oil
- 6 celery stalks
- 2 medium yellow onions
- 1 teaspoon ground cumin
- ½ teaspoon ground cinnamon
- 1 teaspoon ginger powder
- 6 garlic cloves, minced
- ½ teaspoon paprika
- 1 teaspoon salt
- ¼ teaspoon freshly ground black pepper
- 2 cups low-sodium vegetable stock
- 2 medium zucchinis
- 2 cups cauliflower, cut into florets
- 1 medium eggplant
- 1 cup green olives
- 13.5 ounces artichoke hearts
- ½ cup chopped fresh cilantro leaves, for garnish
- ½ cup plain Greek yogurt, for garnish
- ½ cup chopped fresh flat-leaf parsley, for garnish

Direction:

1. Cook olive oil in a stockpot over medium-high heat.

2. Add the celery and onion to the pot and sauté for 6 minutes or until the celery is tender and the onion is translucent.

3. Add the cumin, cinnamon, ginger, garlic, paprika, salt, and black pepper to the pot and sauté for 2 minutes more until aromatic.

4. Pour the vegetable stock to the pot and bring to a boil.

5. Turn down the heat to low, and add the zucchini, cauliflower, and eggplant to the pot. Put the lid on and simmer for 30 minutes or until the vegetables are soft.

6. Then add the olives and artichoke hearts to the pot and simmer for 15 minutes more.

7. Pour them into a large serving bowl or a Tagine, then serve with cilantro, Greek yogurt, and parsley on top.

Nutrition

312 calories

21.2g fat

6.1g protein

6.8g Carbohydrates

23. Citrus Pistachios and Asparagus

Difficulty: Intermediate level

Preparation Time: 10 minutes

Cooking Time: 10 minutes

Serving: 4

Size/ Portion:

Ingredients:

- Zest and juice of 2 clementine
- Zest and juice of 1 lemon

- 1 tablespoon red wine vinegar
- 3 tablespoons extra-virgin olive oil
- 1 teaspoon salt
- ¼ teaspoon black pepper
- ½ cup pistachios, shelled
- 1-pound fresh asparagus
- 1 tablespoon water

Direction:

1. Combine the zest and juice of clementine and lemon, vinegar, 2 tablespoons of olive oil, ½ teaspoon of salt, and black pepper in a bowl. Stir to mix well. Set aside.

2. Toast the pistachios in a nonstick skillet over medium-high heat for 2 minutes or until golden brown. Transfer the roasted pistachios to a clean work surface, then chop roughly. Mix the pistachios with the citrus mixture. Set aside.

3. Heat the remaining olive oil in the nonstick skillet over medium-high heat.

4. Add the asparagus to the skillet and sauté for 2 minutes, then season with remaining salt.

5. Add the water to the skillet. Turn down the heat to low, and put the lid on. Simmer for 4 minutes until the asparagus is tender.

6. Remove the asparagus from the skillet to a large dish. Pour the citrus and pistachios mixture over the asparagus. Toss to coat well before serving.

Nutrition:

211 calories

17.5g fat

5.9g protein

18.6g Carbohydrates

24. Tomato and Parsley Stuffed Eggplant

Difficulty: Intermediate level

Preparation Time: 25 minutes

Cooking Time: 2 hours

Serving: 6

Size/ portion: ½ cup

Ingredients:

- ¼ cup extra-virgin olive oil
- 3 small eggplants, cut in half lengthwise
- 1 teaspoon sea salt
- ½ teaspoon freshly ground black pepper
- 1 large yellow onion, finely chopped
- 4 garlic cloves, minced
- 15 ounces diced tomatoes
- ¼ cup fresh flat-leaf parsley

Direction:

1. Brush insert of the slow cooker with 2 tablespoons of olive oil.

2. Cut some slits on the cut side of each eggplant half, keep a ¼-inch space between each slit.

3. Place the eggplant halves in the slow cooker, skin side down. Sprinkle with salt and black pepper.

4. Cook remaining olive oil in a nonstick skillet over medium-high heat.

5. Add the onion and garlic to the skillet and sauté for 3 minutes or until the onion is translucent.

6. Add the parsley and tomatoes with the juice to the skillet, and sprinkle with salt and black pepper. Sauté for 5 more minutes or until they are tender.

7. Divide and spoon the mixture in the skillet on the eggplant halves.

8. Close and cook on HIGH for 2 hours.

9. Transfer the eggplant to a plate, and allow to cool for a few minutes before serving.

Nutrition:

455 calories

13g fat

14g protein

12g Carbohydrates

25. Ratatouille

Difficulty: Professional level

Preparation Time: 15 minutes

Cooking Time: 7 hours

Serving: 6

Size/ Portion: 2 ounces

Ingredient:

- 3 tablespoons extra-virgin olive oil
- 1 large eggplant
- 2 large onions
- 4 small zucchinis
- 2 green bell peppers
- 6 large tomatoes
- 2 tablespoons fresh flat-leaf parsley
- 1 teaspoon dried basil
- 2 garlic cloves, minced
- 2 teaspoons sea salt
- ¼ teaspoon black pepper

Direction

1. Grease insert of the slow cooker with 2 tablespoons olive oil.

2. Arrange the vegetables slices, strips, and wedges alternately in the insert of the slow cooker.

3. Spread the parsley on top of the vegetables, and season with basil, garlic, salt, and black pepper. Drizzle with the remaining olive oil.

4. Cover on and cook on LOW for 7 hours until the vegetables are tender.

5. Transfer the vegetables on a plate and serve warm.

Nutrition:

265 calories 1.7g fat

8.3g protein 9.8g Carbohydrates

26. Gemista

Difficulty: Professional level

Preparation Time: 15 minutes

Cooking Time: 4 hours

Serving: 4

Size/ portion: 2 ounces

Ingredients:

- 2 tablespoons extra-virgin olive oil
- 4 large bell peppers, any color
- ½ cup uncooked couscous
- 1 teaspoon oregano
- 1 garlic clove, minced
- 1 cup crumbled feta cheese
- 1 (15-ounce) can cannellini beans
- 4 green onions

Direction:

1. Brush insert of the slow cooker with 2 tablespoons olive oil.

2. Cut a ½-inch slice below the stem from the top of the bell pepper. Discard the stem only and chop the sliced top portion under the stem, and reserve in a bowl. Hollow the bell pepper with a spoon.

3. Mix remaining ingredients, except for the green parts of the green onion and lemon wedges, to the bowl of chopped bell pepper top. Stir to mix well.

4. Spoon the mixture in the hollowed bell pepper, and arrange the stuffed bell

peppers in the slow cooker, then drizzle with more olive oil.

5. Close and cook at HIGH for 4 hours or until the bell peppers are soft.

6. Remove the bell peppers from the slow cooker and serve on a plate. Sprinkle with green parts of the green onions, and squeeze the lemon wedges on top before serving.

Nutrition:

246 calories 9g fat

11.1g protein 6.7g Carbohydrates

27.   Stuffed Cabbage Rolls

Difficulty: Professional level

Preparation Time: 15 minutes

Cooking Time: 2 hours

Serving: 4

Size/ Portion: 1 roll

Ingredients:

- 4 tablespoons olive oil
- 1 large head green cabbage
- 1 large yellow onion
- 3 ounces (85 g) feta cheese
- ½ cup dried currants
- 3 cups cooked pearl barley
- 2 tablespoons fresh flat-leaf parsley
- 2 tablespoons pine nuts, toasted
- ½ teaspoon sea salt
- ½ teaspoon black pepper
- 15 ounces (425 g) crushed tomatoes, with the juice
- ½ cup apple juice
- 1 tablespoon apple cider vinegar

Direction:

1. Rub insert of the slow cooker with 2 tablespoons olive oil.

2. Blanch the cabbage in a pot of water for 8 minutes. Remove it from the water, and allow to cool, then separate 16 leaves from the cabbage. Set aside.

3. Drizzle the remaining olive oil in a nonstick skillet, and heat over medium heat.

4. Sauté onion for 6 minutes. Transfer the onion to a bowl.

5. Add the feta cheese, currants, barley, parsley, and pine nuts to the bowl of cooked onion, then sprinkle with ¼ teaspoon of salt and ¼ teaspoon of black pepper.

6. Arrange the cabbage leaves on a clean work surface. Spoon 1/3 cup of the mixture on the center of each leaf, then fold the edge of the leaf over the mixture and roll it up. Place the cabbage rolls in the slow cooker, seam side down.

7. Combine the remaining ingredients in a separate bowl, then pour the mixture over the cabbage rolls.

8. Close and cook in HIGH for 2 hours.

9. Remove the cabbage rolls from the slow cooker and serve warm.

Nutrition: 383 calories 17g fat

11g protein 14g Carbohydrates

28.   Brussels Sprouts with Balsamic Glaze

Difficulty: Professional level

Preparation Time: 15 minutes

Cooking Time: 2 hours

Serving: 6

Size/ Portion: 1 lb.

Balsamic glaze:

- 1 cup balsamic vinegar
- ¼ cup honey

Other:

- 2 tablespoons extra-virgin olive oil

- 2 pounds (907 g) Brussels sprouts
- 2 cups low-sodium vegetable soup
- 1 teaspoon sea salt
- Freshly ground black pepper, to taste
- ¼ cup Parmesan cheese, grated
- ¼ cup pine nuts, toasted

Direction:

1. Brush insert of the slow cooker with olive oil.
2. Make the balsamic glaze: Combine the balsamic vinegar and honey in a saucepan. Stir to mix well. Over medium-high heat, bring to a boil. Turn down the heat to low, then simmer for 20 minutes or until the glaze reduces in half and has a thick consistency.
3. Put the Brussels sprouts, vegetable soup, and ½ teaspoon of salt in the slow cooker, stir to combine.
4. Cover and cook at HIGH for 2 hours.
5. Transfer the Brussels sprouts to a plate, and sprinkle the remaining salt and black pepper to season. Drizzle the balsamic glaze over the Brussels sprouts, then serve with Parmesan and pine nuts.

Nutrition: 270 calories

11g fat 8.7g protein 9.7g Carbohydrates

29. Spinach Salad with Citrus Vinaigrette

Difficulty: Professional level

Preparation Time: 10 minutes

Cooking Time: 0 minutes

Servings: 4

Size/ portion: 2 cups

Ingredients:

Citrus Vinaigrette:

- ¼ cup extra-virgin olive oil
- 3 tablespoons balsamic vinegar

- ½ teaspoon fresh lemon zest
- ½ teaspoon salt

SALAD:

- 1-pound (454 g) baby spinach
- 1 large ripe tomato
- 1 medium red onion

Direction:

1. Make the citrus vinaigrette: Stir together the olive oil, balsamic vinegar, lemon zest, and salt in a bowl until mixed well.
2. Make the salad: Place the baby spinach, tomato and onions in a separate salad bowl. Drizzle the citrus vinaigrette over the salad and gently toss until the vegetables are coated thoroughly.

Nutrition:

173 Calories

14g fat

4.1g protein

3.4g Carbohydrates

30. Kale Salad with Pistachio and Parmesan

Difficulty: Professional level

Preparation Time: 20 minutes

Cooking Time: 0 minutes

Serving: 6

Size/ Portion: 2 cups

Ingredients:

- 6 cups raw kale
- ¼ cup extra-virgin olive oil
- 2 tablespoons lemon juice
- ½ teaspoon smoked paprika
- 2 cups chopped arugula
- 1/3 cup unsalted pistachios
- 6 tablespoons Parmesan cheese

Direction:

1. Put the kale, olive oil, lemon juice, and paprika in a large bowl. Using your hands to massage the sauce into the kale until coated completely. Allow the kale to marinate for about 10 minutes.

2. When ready to serve, add the arugula and pistachios into the bowl of kale. Toss well and divide the salad into six salad bowls. Serve sprinkled with 1 tablespoon shredded Parmesan cheese.

Nutrition:

106 Calories

9.2g fat

4.2g protein

5.7g Carbohydrates

31. Israeli Eggplant, Chickpea, and Mint Sauté

Difficulty: Intermediate level

Preparation Time: 5 minutes

Cooking Time: 20 minutes

Serving: 6

Size/ Portion: 2 cups

Ingredients:

- 1 medium globe eggplant
- 1 tablespoon extra-virgin olive oil
- 2 tablespoons lemon juice
- 2 tablespoons balsamic vinegar
- 1 teaspoon ground cumin
- ¼ teaspoon salt
- 1 (15-ounce) can chickpeas
- 1 cup sliced sweet onion
- ¼ cup mint leaves
- 1 tablespoon sesame seeds
- 1 garlic clove

Direction:

1. Place one oven rack about 4 inches below the broiler element. Turn the broiler to the highest setting to preheat. Grease rimmed baking sheet using nonstick cooking spray.

2. Slice eggplant lengthwise into four slabs (½- to 5/8-inch thick). Place the eggplant slabs on the prepared baking sheet. Put aside.

3. Scourge oil, lemon juice, vinegar, cumin, and salt. Brush 2 tablespoons of the lemon dressing over both sides of the eggplant slabs.

4. Broil the eggplant under the heating element for 4 minutes, flip them, and then broil for 4 minutes.

5. While the eggplant is broiling, combine the chickpeas, onion, mint, sesame seeds, and garlic. Add the reserved dressing, and gently mix.

6. When done, situate slabs from the baking sheet to a cooling rack and cool for 3 minutes. When slightly cooled, cut each slab crosswise into ½-inch strips.

7. Toss eggplant to the mixture and serve warm.

Nutrition:

159 Calories

4g Fat

6g Protein

8g Carbohydrates

32. Mediterranean Lentils and Rice

Difficulty: Professional level

Preparation Time: 5 minutes

Cooking Time: 25 minutes

Serving: 4

Size/ Portion: 2 cups

Ingredients:

- 2¼ cups low-sodium vegetable broth

- ½ cup lentils
- ½ cup uncooked instant brown rice
- ½ cup diced carrots
- ½ cup diced celery
- 1 (2.25-ounce) can sliced olives
- ¼ cup diced red onion
- ¼ cup chopped fresh curly-leaf parsley
- 1½ tablespoons extra-virgin olive oil
- 1 tablespoon freshly squeezed lemon juice
- 1 garlic clove
- ¼ teaspoon kosher or sea salt
- ¼ teaspoon black pepper

Direction:

1. Position saucepan over high heat, bring the broth and lentils to a boil, cover, and lower the heat to medium-low. Cook for 8 minutes.

2. Raise the heat to medium, and stir in the rice. Cover the pot and cook the mixture for 15 minutes. Take away pot from the heat and let it sit, covered, for 1 minute, then stir.

3. While the lentils and rice are cooking, mix together the carrots, celery, olives, onion, and parsley in a large serving bowl.

4. In a small bowl, whisk together the oil, lemon juice, garlic, salt, and pepper. Set aside.

5. When cooked, put them to the serving bowl. Pour the dressing on top, and mix everything together. Serve.

Nutrition:

230 Calories

8g Fat

8g Protein

9g Carbohydrates

33. Brown Rice Pilaf with Golden Raisins

Difficulty: Professional level

Preparation Time: 5 minutes

Cooking Time: 15 minutes

Serving: 6

Size/ Portion: 2 cups

Ingredients:

- 1 tablespoon extra-virgin olive oil
- 1 cup chopped onion
- ½ cup shredded carrot
- 1 teaspoon ground cumin
- ½ teaspoon ground cinnamon
- 2 cups instant brown rice
- 1¾ cups 100% orange juice
- ¼ cup water
- 1 cup golden raisins
- ½ cup shelled pistachios

Direction:

1. Put saucepan on medium-high heat, cook onion for 5 minutes. Sauté carrot, cumin, and cinnamon. Stir in the rice, orange juice, and water. Bring to a boil, cover, then lower the heat to medium-low. Simmer for 7 minutes.

2. Stir in the raisins, pistachios, and chives (if using) and serve.

Nutrition: 320 Calories 7g Fat

6g Protein 8g Carbohydrates

34. Chinese Soy Eggplant

Difficulty: Intermediate level

Preparation Time: 5 Minutes

Cooking Time: 10 Minutes

Servings: 2

Ingredients:

- Four tablespoons coconut oil

- Two eggplants, sliced into 3-inch in length
- Four cloves of garlic, minced
- One onion, chopped
- One teaspoon ginger, grated
- ¼ cup coconut aminos
- One teaspoon lemon juice, freshly squeezed

Directions:

1. Heat oil in a pot.
2. Pan-fry the eggplants for minutes on all sides.
3. Add the garlic and onions until fragrant, around minutes.
4. Stir in the ginger, coconut aminos, and lemon juice.
5. Add a ½ cup of water and let it simmer. Cook until eggplant is tender.

Nutrition:

Calories per **Serving:** 409

Carbs: 40.8g

Protein: 6.6g

Fat: 28.3g

35.   Cauliflower Mash

Difficulty: Intermediate level

Preparation Time:5 Minutes

Cooking Time:0 Minutes

Servings:2

Ingredients:

- Crushed red pepper to taste
- 1 tsp fresh thyme
- 2 tsp chopped chives
- 2 tbsp. nutritional yeast
- 2 tbsp. filtered water
- One garlic clove, peeled
- One lemon, juice extracted
- ¼ cup pine nuts
- 3 cups cauliflower, chopped

Directions:

1. Mix all fixings in a blender or food processor. Pulse until smooth.

2. Scoop into a bowl and add crushed red peppers.

Nutrition:

Calories per **Serving:** 224

Carbs: 19.8g

Protein: 10.5g

Fat: 13.6g

36.   Vegetarian Cabbage Rolls

Difficulty: Intermediate level

Preparation Time:5 Minutes

Cooking Time:1 Hour and 30 Minutes

Servings:2

Ingredients:

- One large head green cabbage
- 1 cup long-grain rice, rinsed
- Two medium zucchinis, finely diced
- 4 TB. minced garlic
- 2 tsp. salt
- 1 tsp. ground black pepper
- 4 cups plain tomato sauce
- 2 cups of water
- 1 tsp. dried mint

Directions:

1. Cut around a core of cabbage with a knife, and remove the core. Put cabbage, with core side down, in a large, 3-quart pot. Cover cabbage with water, set over high heat, and cook for 30 minutes. Drain cabbage, set aside to cool, and separate leaves. (You need 24 leaves.)
2. In a large bowl, combine long-grain rice, zucchini, one tablespoon garlic, one teaspoon salt, and 1/teaspoon black pepper.
3. In a 2-quart pot, combine tomato sauce, water, remaining tablespoons garlic, mint, remaining one teaspoon salt, and 1/2 teaspoon black pepper.
4. Lay each cabbage leaf flat on your work surface, spoon two tablespoons filling each leaf, and roll leaf. Layer rolls in a large pot, pour the sauce into the pot,

cover, and cook over medium-low heat for 1 hour.

5. Let rolls sit for 20 minutes before serving warm with Greek yogurt.

Nutrition:

Calories per **Serving:** 120 Carbs: 8.0g

Protein: 2.3g Fat: 9.5g

37. Vegan Sesame Tofu and Eggplants

Difficulty: Intermediate level

Preparation Time: 5 Minutes

Cooking Time: 15 Minutes

Servings: 4

Ingredients:

- Five tablespoons olive oil
- 1-pound firm tofu, sliced
- Three tablespoons rice vinegar
- Two teaspoons Swerve sweetener
- Two whole eggplants, sliced
- ¼ cup of soy sauce
- Salt and pepper to taste
- Four tablespoons toasted sesame oil
- ¼ cup sesame seeds
- 1 cup fresh cilantro, chopped

Directions:

1. Heat the oil in a pan for 2 minutes.
2. Pan-fry the tofu for 3 minutes on each side.
3. Stir in the rice vinegar, sweetener, eggplants, and soy sauce—season with salt and pepper to taste.
4. Close the lid, then cook for around 5 minutes on medium fire. Stir and continue cooking for another 5 minutes.
5. Toss in the sesame oil, sesame seeds, and cilantro.
6. Serve and enjoy.

Nutrition:

Calories per **Serving:** 616

Carbs: 27.4g Protein: 23.9g

Fat: 49.2g

38. Steamed Squash Chowder

Difficulty: Intermediate level

Preparation Time: 5 Minutes

Cooking Time: 40 Minutes

Servings: 4

Ingredients:

- 3 cups chicken broth
- 2 tbsp. ghee
- 1 tsp chili powder
- ½ tsp cumin
- 1 ½ tsp salt
- 2 tsp cinnamon
- 3 tbsp. olive oil
- Two carrots, chopped
- One small yellow onion, chopped
- One green apple, sliced and cored
- One large butternut squash

Directions:

1. In a large pot on medium-high fire, melt ghee.
2. Once the ghee is hot, sauté onions for 5 minutes or until soft and translucent.
3. Add olive oil, chili powder, cumin, salt, and cinnamon. Sauté for half a minute.
4. Add chopped squash and apples.
5. Sauté for 10 minutes while stirring once in a while.
6. Add broth, cover, and cook on medium fire for twenty minutes or until apples and squash are tender.
7. With an immersion blender, puree the chowder. Adjust consistency by adding more water.
8. Add more salt or pepper depending on desire.
9. Serve and enjoy.

Nutrition:

Calories per **Serving:** 228

Carbs: 17.9g

Protein: 2.2g

Fat: 18.0g

39.   Collard Green Wrap Greek Style

Difficulty: Professional level

Preparation Time:5 Minutes

Cooking Time:0 Minutes

Servings:4

Ingredients:

- ½ block feta, cut into 4 (1-inch thick) strips (4-oz)
- ½ cup purple onion, diced
- ½ medium red bell pepper, julienned
- One medium cucumber, julienned
- Four large cherry tomatoes halved
- Four large collard green leaves washed
- Eight whole kalamata olives halved
- 1 cup full-fat plain Greek yogurt
- One tablespoon white vinegar
- One teaspoon garlic powder
- Two tablespoons minced fresh dill
- Two tablespoons olive oil
- 2.5-ounces cucumber, seeded and grated (¼-whole)
- Salt and pepper to taste

Directions:

1. Make the Tzatziki sauce first: make sure to squeeze out all the excess liquid from the cucumber after grating. In a small bowl, mix all sauce fixings thoroughly and refrigerate.
2. Prepare and slice all wrap ingredients.
3. On a flat surface, spread one collard green leaf. Spread two tablespoons of Tzatziki sauce in the middle of the leaf.
4. Layer ¼ of each of the tomatoes, feta, olives, onion, pepper, and cucumber. Place them on the center of the leaf, like piling them high instead of spreading them.
5. Fold the leaf like you would a burrito. Repeat process for remaining ingredients.
6. Serve and enjoy.

Nutrition:

Calories per **Serving:** 165.3

Protein: 7.0g Carbs: 9.9g Fat: 11.2g

40.   Cayenne Eggplant Spread

Difficulty: Professional level

Preparation Time:5 Minutes

Cooking Time:50 Minutes

Servings:4

Ingredients:

- Two eggplants, trimmed
- One teaspoon cayenne pepper
- One teaspoon salt
- ½ teaspoon harissa
- One tablespoon sesame oil
- Three tablespoons Plain yogurt
- One garlic clove, peeled
- 1/3 teaspoon sumac
- One teaspoon ground paprika
- One teaspoon lemon juice

Directions:

1. Cut the eggplants on the halves and rub them with salt.
2. Preheat the oven to 375F.
3. Arrange the eggplant halves in the tray and bake them for 50 minutes.
4. When the eggplants are soft, they are ready to be used.
5. Peel the eggplants and put the peeled eggplant pulp in the blender.
6. Add cayenne pepper, harissa, sesame oil, Plain yogurt, garlic clove, sumac, and lemon juice.
7. Blend the mixture until smooth and soft.
8. Transfer the cooked meal to the serving bowls and sprinkle with ground paprika.

Nutrition:

Calories 113

Fat 4.3

Fiber 10

Carbs 18

Protein 3.6

41.   Cilantro Potato Mash

Difficulty: Professional level

Preparation Time: 5 Minutes

Cooking Time: 20 Minutes

Servings: 2

Ingredients:

- 1 cup yam, chopped
- One tablespoon cream
- ½ teaspoon dried cilantro
- 1 cup of water
- ½ teaspoon salt

Directions:

1. Boil yum in water for 20 minutes or until it is soft.
2. Then drain the water and mash the yam with the help of the potato masher.
3. Add cream dried cilantro, and salt.
4. Mix up well.

Nutrition:

Calories 92

Fat 0.5

Fiber 3.1

Carbs 21.1

Protein 1.2

42.   Cheese and Broccoli Balls

Difficulty: Professional level

Preparation Time: 5 Minutes

Cooking Time: 5 Minutes

Servings: 4

Ingredients:

- ¾ cup almond flour
- Two large eggs
- Two teaspoons baking powder
- 4 ounces fresh broccoli
- 4 ounces mozzarella cheese
- Seven tablespoons flaxseed meal
- Salt and Pepper to taste
- ¼ cup fresh chopped dill
- ¼ cup mayonnaise

- ½ tablespoon lemon juice
- Salt and pepper to taste

Directions:

1. Place broccoli in the food processor and pulse into small pieces. Transfer to a bowl.
2. Add ¼ cup flaxseed meal, baking powder, almond flour, and cheese. Season with pepper and salt if desired. Mix well—place remaining flaxseed meal in a small bowl.
3. Add eggs and combine thoroughly. Roll the batter into 1-inch balls. Then roll in flaxseed meal to hide the balls.
4. Cook balls in a 375oF deep-fryer until golden brown, about 5 minutes. Transfer cooked balls on to a paper towel-lined plate.
5. In the meantime, make the sauce by combining all fixings in a medium bowl.
6. Serve cheese and broccoli balls with the plunging sauce on the side.

Nutrition:

Calories per **Serving:** 312

Protein: 18.4g

Carbs: 9.6g

Fat: 23.2g

43.   Hot Pepper Sauce

Difficulty: Professional level

Preparation Time: 10 Minutes

Cooking Time: 20 Minutes

Servings: 4 Cups

Ingredients:

- Two red hot fresh chiles, deseeded
- Two dried chiles
- Two garlic cloves, peeled
- ½ small yellow onion, roughly chopped
- 2 cups of water
- 2 cups white vinegar

Directions:

1. Place all the fixings except the vinegar in a medium saucepan over medium heat.

Allow simmering for 20 minutes until softened.

2. Transfer the combination to a food processor or blender. Stir in the vinegar and pulse until very smooth.

3. Serve instantly or transfer to a sealed container and refrigerate for up to 3 months.

Nutrition:

Calories: 20

Fat: 1.2g

Protein: 0.6g

Carbs: 4.4g

Fiber: 0.6g

Sodium: 12mg

44. Avocado Gazpacho

Difficulty: Professional level

Preparation Time: 15 minutes

Cooking Time: 0 minute

Serving: 4

Size/ portion: 2 cups

Ingredients:

- 2 cups chopped tomatoes
- 2 large ripe avocados
- 1 large cucumber
- 1 medium bell pepper
- 1 cup plain whole-milk Greek yogurt
- ¼ cup extra-virgin olive oil
- ¼ cup chopped fresh cilantro
- ¼ cup chopped scallions
- 2 tablespoons red wine vinegar
- Juice of 2 limes or 1 lemon
- ½ to 1 teaspoon salt
- ¼ teaspoon black pepper

Direction:

1. In a blender or in a large bowl, if using an immersion blender, combine the tomatoes, avocados, cucumber, bell pepper, yogurt, olive oil, and cilantro, scallions, vinegar, and lime juice. Blend until smooth. If using a stand blender, you may need to blend in two or three batches.

2. Season with salt and pepper and blend to combine the flavors.

3. Chill for 2 hours before serving. Serve cold.

Nutrition:

392 Calories

32g Fat

6g Protein

8g Carbohydrates

45. Roasted Garlic Hummus

Difficulty: Professional level

Preparation Time: 9 minutes

Cooking Time: 33 minutes

Serving: 4

Size/ Portion: 2 tablespoons

Ingredients:

- 1 cup dried chickpeas
- 4 cups water
- 1 tablespoon plus ¼ cup extra-virgin olive oil, divided
- 1/3 cup tahini
- 1 teaspoon ground cumin
- ½ teaspoon onion powder
- ¾ teaspoon salt
- ½ teaspoon ground black pepper
- 1/3 cup lemon juice
- 3 tablespoons mashed roasted garlic
- 2 tablespoons chopped fresh parsley

Direction:

1. Situate chickpeas, water, and 1 tablespoon oil in the Instant Pot®.

Cover, press steam release to Sealing, set Manual button, and time to 30 minutes.

2. When the timer beeps, quick-release the pressure. Select Cancel button and open. Strain, reserving the cooking liquid.

3. Place chickpeas, remaining ¼ cup oil, tahini, cumin, onion powder, salt, pepper, lemon juice, and roasted garlic in a food processor and process until creamy. Top with parsley. Serve at room temperature.

Nutrition

104 Calories

6g Fat

4g Protein

7g Carbohydrates

Lunch and Dinner (Poultry and Meat Recipes)

1. Chicken and Olives

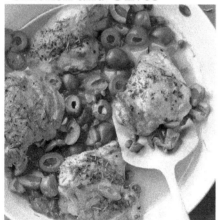

Difficulty: Novice level

Preparation Time: 10 minutes

Cooking Time: 15 minutes

Servings: 4

Ingredients:

- 4 chicken breasts, skinless and boneless
- 2 tablespoons garlic, minced
- 1 tablespoon oregano, dried
- Salt and black pepper to the taste
- 2 tablespoons olive oil
- ½ cup chicken stock
- Juice of 1 lemon
- 1 cup red onion, chopped
- 1 and ½ cups tomatoes, cubed
- ¼ cup green olives, pitted and sliced
- A handful parsley, chopped

Directions:

1. Heat up a pan w/ the oil over medium-high heat, add the chicken, garlic, salt and pepper and brown for 2 minutes on each side.

2. Add the rest of the ingredients, toss, bring the mix to a simmer and cook over medium heat for 13 minutes.

3. Divide the mix between plates and serve.

Nutrition:

Calories 135, Fat 5.8, Fiber 3.4,

Carbs 12.1, Protein 9.6

2. Chicken Bake

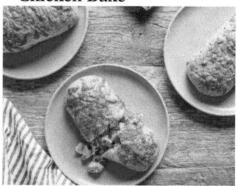

Difficulty: Novice level

Preparation Time: 10 minutes

Cooking Time: 30 minutes

Servings: 4

Ingredients:

- 1 and ½ pounds chicken thighs, skinless, boneless and cubed
- 2 garlic cloves, minced
- 1 tablespoon oregano, chopped
- 2 tablespoons olive oil
- 1 tablespoon red wine vinegar

- ½ cup canned artichokes, drained and chopped
- 1 red onion, sliced
- 1 pound whole wheat fusili pasta, cooked
- ½ cup canned white beans, drained and rinsed
- ½ cup parsley, chopped
- 1 cup mozzarella, shredded
- Salt and black pepper to the taste

Directions:

1. Heat up a pan with half of the oil over medium-high heat, add the meat and brown for 5 minutes.
2. Grease a baking pan with the rest of the oil, add the browned chicken, and the rest of the ingredients except the pasta and the mozzarella.
3. Spread the pasta all over and toss gently.
4. Now, sprinkle the mozzarella on top and bake at 425 degrees F for 25 minutes.
5. Divide the bake between plates and serve.

Nutrition: Calories 195, Fat 5.8, Fiber 3.4,

Carbs 12.1, Protein 11.6

3. Pesto Chicken Mix

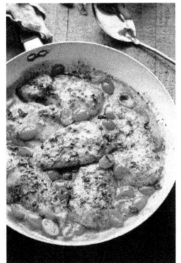

Difficulty: Novice level

Preparation Time: 10 minutes

Cooking Time: 40 minutes

Servings: 4

Ingredients:

- 4 chicken breast halves, skinless and boneless
- 3 tomatoes, cubed
- 1 cup mozzarella, shredded
- ½ cup basil pesto
- A pinch of salt and black pepper
- Cooking spray

Directions:

1. Grease a baking dish lined with parchment paper with the cooking spray.
2. In a bowl, mix the chicken with salt, pepper and the pesto and rub well.
3. Place the chicken on the baking sheet, top with tomatoes and shredded mozzarella and bake at 400 degrees F for 40 mins.
4. Divide the mix between plates & serve with a side salad.

Nutrition:

Calories 341, Fat 20, Fiber 1,

Carbs 4, Protein 32

4. Chicken Wrap

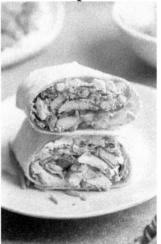

Difficulty: Novice level

Preparation Time: 10 minutes

Cooking Time: 0 minutes

Servings: 2

Ingredients:

- 2 whole wheat tortilla flatbreads

- 6 chicken breast slices, skinless, boneless, cooked and shredded
- A handful baby spinach
- 2 provolone cheese slices
- 4 tomato slices
- 10 kalamata olives, pitted and sliced
- 1 red onion, sliced
- 2 tablespoons roasted peppers, chopped

Directions:

1. Arrange the tortillas on a working surface, and divide the chicken and the other ingredients on each.
2. Roll the tortillas and serve them right away.

Nutrition:

Calories 190,

Fat 6.8,

Fiber 3.5,

Carbs 15.1,

Protein 6.6

5.   Chicken and Artichokes

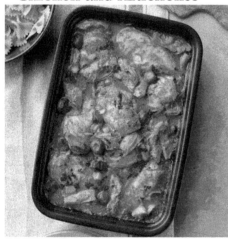

Difficulty: Novice level

Preparation Time: 10 minutes

Cooking Time: 20 minutes

Servings: 4

Ingredients:

- 2 pounds chicken breast, skinless, boneless and sliced

- A pinch of salt and black pepper
- 4 tablespoons olive oil
- 8 ounces canned roasted artichoke hearts, drained
- 6 ounces sun-dried tomatoes, chopped
- 3 tablespoons capers, drained
- 2 tablespoons lemon juice

Directions:

1. Heat up a pan with half of the oil over medium-high heat, add the artichokes and the other ingredients except the chicken, stir and sauté for 10 minutes.
2. Transfer the mix to a bowl, heat up the pan again with the rest of the oil over medium-high heat, add the meat and cook for 4 minutes on each side.
3. Return the veggie mix to the pan, toss, cook everything for 2-3 minutes more, divide between plates and serve.

Nutrition:

Calories 552,

Fat 28,

Fiber 6,

Carbs 33,

Protein 43

6.   Chicken Kebabs

Difficulty: Novice level

Preparation Time: 30 minutes

Cooking Time: 20 minutes

Servings: 4

Ingredients:

- 2 chicken breasts, skinless, boneless and cubed
- 1 red bell pepper, cut into squares
- 1 red onion, roughly cut into squares
- 2 teaspoons sweet paprika
- 1 teaspoon nutmeg, ground
- 1 teaspoon Italian seasoning
- ¼ teaspoon smoked paprika
- A pinch of salt and black pepper
- ¼ teaspoon cardamom, ground

- Juice of 1 lemon
- 3 garlic cloves, minced
- ½ cup olive oil

Directions:

1. Combine the chicken with the onion, the bell pepper and the other ingredients, toss well, cover the bowl and keep in the fridge for 30 minutes.
2. Assemble skewers with chicken, peppers and the onions, place them on your preheated grill and cook over medium heat for 8 minutes on each side.
3. Divide the kebabs between plates and serve with a side salad.

Nutrition:

Calories 262,

Fat 14,

Fiber 2,

Carbs 14,

Protein 20

7. Rosemary Pork Chops

Difficulty: Novice level

Preparation Time: 10 minutes

Cooking Time: 35 minutes

Servings: 4

Ingredients:

- 4 pork loin chops, boneless
- Salt and black pepper to the taste
- 4 garlic cloves, minced
- 1 tablespoon rosemary, chopped
- 1 tablespoon olive oil

Directions:

1. In a roasting pan, combine the pork chops with the rest of the ingredients, toss, and bake at 425 degrees F for 10 min.
2. Low the heat to 350 degrees F and cook the chops for 25 minutes more.
3. Divide the chops between plates and serve with a side salad.

Nutrition:

Calories 161,

Fat 5,

Fiber 1,

Carbs 1,

Protein 25

8. Pork Chops and Relish

Difficulty: Novice level

Preparation Time: 15 minutes

Cooking Time: 14 minutes

Servings: 6

Ingredients:

- 6 pork chops, boneless
- 7 ounces marinated artichoke hearts, chopped and their liquid reserved
- A pinch of salt and black pepper
- 1 teaspoon hot pepper sauce
- 1 and ½ cups tomatoes, cubed
- 1 jalapeno pepper, chopped
- ½ cup roasted bell peppers, chopped
- ½ cup black olives, pitted and sliced

Directions:

1. In a bowl, mix the chops with the pepper sauce, reserved liquid from the artichokes, cover and keep in the fridge for 15 minutes.
2. Heat up a grill over medium-high heat, add the pork chops and cook for 7 minutes on each side.
3. In a bowl, combine the artichokes with the peppers and the remaining ingredients, toss, divide on top of the chops and serve.

Nutrition:

Calories 215,

Fat 6,

Fiber 1,

Carbs 6,

Protein 35

9. Pork Chops and Peach Chutney

Difficulty: Intermediate level

Preparation Time: 10 minutes

Cooking Time: 30 minutes

Servings: 4

Ingredients:

- 4 pork loin chops, boneless
- Salt and black pepper to the taste
- ½ teaspoon garlic powder
- ¼ teaspoon cumin, ground
- ½ teaspoon sage, dried
- Cooking spray
- 1 teaspoon chili powder
- 1 teaspoon oregano, dried

For the chutney:

- ¼ cup shallot, minced
- 1 teaspoon olive oil
- 2 cups peaches, peeled and chopped
- ½ cup red sweet pepper, chopped
- 2 tablespoons jalapeno chili pepper, minced
- 1 tablespoon balsamic vinegar
- ½ teaspoon cinnamon powder
- 2 tablespoons cilantro, chopped

Directions:

1. Heat up a pan w/ the olive oil over medium heat, add the shallot and sauté for 5 minutes.
2. Add the sweet pepper, peaches, chili pepper, vinegar, cinnamon and the cilantro, stir, simmer for 10 minutes and take off the heat.
3. Meanwhile, in a bowl, combine the pork chops with cooking spray, salt, pepper, garlic powder, cumin, sage, oregano and chili powder and rub well.
4. Heat up your grill over medium-high heat, add pork chops, cook for 6-7 minutes on each side, divide between plates and serve with the chutney on top.

Nutrition:

Calories 297, Fat 10, Fiber 2,

Carbs 13, Protein 38

10. Glazed Pork Chops

Difficulty: Intermediate level

Preparation Time: 10 minutes

Cooking Time: 20 minutes

Servings: 4

Ingredients:

- ¼ cup apricot preserves
- 4 pork chops, boneless
- 1 tablespoon thyme, chopped
- ½ teaspoon cinnamon powder
- 2 tablespoons olive oil

Directions:

1. Heat up a pan w/ the oil over medium-high heat, add the apricot preserves and cinnamon, whisk, bring to a simmer, cook for 10 minutes and take off the heat.
2. Heat up your grill over medium-high heat, brush the pork chops with some of the apricot glaze, place them on the grill and cook for 10 minutes.
3. Flip the chops, brush them with more apricot glaze, cook for 10 minutes more and divide between plates.
4. Sprinkle the thyme on top and serve.

Nutrition:

Calories 225,

Fat 11,

Fiber 0,

Carbs 6,

Protein 23

11. Pork Chops and Cherries Mix

Difficulty: Intermediate level

Preparation Time: 10 minutes

Cooking Time: 12 minutes

Servings: 4

Ingredients:

- 4 pork chops, boneless
- Salt and black pepper to the taste
- ½ cup cranberry juice

- 1 and ½ teaspoons spicy mustard
- ½ cup dark cherries, pitted and halved
- Cooking spray

Directions:

1. Heat up a pan greased with the cooking spray over medium-high heat, add the pork chops, cook them for 5 minutes on each side and divide between plates.
2. Heat up the same pan over medium heat, add the cranberry juice and the rest of the ingredients, whisk, bring to a simmer, cook for 2 minutes, drizzle over the pork chops and serve.

Nutrition:

Calories 262, Fat 8, Fiber 1,

Carbs 16, Protein 30

12. Baked Pork Chops

Difficulty: Intermediate level

Preparation Time: 10 minutes

Cooking Time: 30 minutes

Servings: 4

Ingredients:

- 4 pork loin chops, boneless
- A pinch of salt and black pepper
- 1 tablespoon sweet paprika
- 2 tablespoons Dijon mustard
- Cooking spray

Directions:

1. In a bowl, mix the pork chops with salt, pepper, paprika and the mustard and rub well.
2. Grease a baking sheet with cooking spray, add the pork chops, cover with tin foil, introduce in the oven and bake at 400 degrees F for 30 minutes.
3. Divide the pork chops between plates and serve with a side salad.

Nutrition:

Calories 167, Fat 5, Fiber 0, Carbs 2, Protein 25

Lunch and Dinner (Salad Recipes)

1. Peppers and Lentils Salad

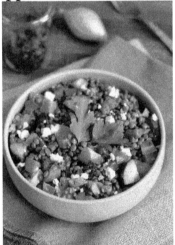

Difficulty: Novice level

Preparation Time: 10 minutes

Cooking Time: 0 minutes

Servings: 4

Size/ Portion: 2 cups

Ingredients:

- 14 ounces canned lentils
- 2 spring onions
- 1 red bell pepper
- 1 green bell pepper
- 1 tablespoon fresh lime juice
- 1/3 cup coriander
- 2 teaspoon balsamic vinegar

Directions:

1. In a salad bowl, combine the lentils with the onions, bell peppers, and the rest of the ingredients, toss and serve.

Nutrition:

200 Calories

2.45g Fat

5.6g Protein

4.3g Carbohydrates

2. Cashews and Red Cabbage Salad

Difficulty: Novice level

Preparation Time: 10 minutes

Cooking Time: 0 minutes

Servings: 4

Size/ Portion: 2 cups

Ingredients:

- 1-pound red cabbage, shredded
- 2 tablespoons coriander, chopped
- ½ cup cashews halved
- 2 tablespoons olive oil
- 1 tomato, cubed
- A pinch of salt and black pepper
- 1 tablespoon white vinegar

Directions:

1. Mix the cabbage with the coriander and the rest of the ingredients in a salad bowl, toss and serve cold.

Nutrition:

210 Calories

6.3g Fat

8g Protein

7g Carbohydrates

3. Tuscan Kale Salad with Anchovies

Difficulty: Professional level

Preparation Time: 45 minutes

Cooking Time: 0 minute

Serving: 4

Size/ Portion: 2 cups

Ingredients:

- 1 large bunch Lacinato
- ¼ cup toasted pine nuts
- 1 cup Parmesan cheese
- ¼ cup extra-virgin olive oil
- 8 anchovy fillets
- 2 to 3 tablespoons lemon juice
- 2 teaspoons red pepper flakes (optional)

Direction:

1. Remove the rough center stems from the kale leaves and roughly tear each leaf into about 4-by-1-inch strips. Situate torn kale in a large bowl and add the pine nuts and cheese.

2. Blend the olive oil, anchovies, lemon juice, and red pepper flakes (if using). Drizzle over the salad and toss to coat well. Let sit at room temperature 30 minutes before serving, tossing again just prior to serving.

Nutrition: 337 Calories 25g Fat 16g Protein

18g Carbohydrates

4. Apples and Pomegranate Salad

Difficulty: Novice level

Preparation Time: 10 minutes

Cooking Time: 0 minutes

Servings: 4

Size/ Portion: 2 cups

Ingredients:

- 3 big apples, cored and cubed
- 1 cup pomegranate seeds
- 3 cups baby arugula
- 1 cup walnuts, chopped
- 1 tablespoon olive oil
- 1 teaspoon white sesame seeds
- 2 tablespoons apple cider vinegar

Directions:

1. Mix the apples with the arugula and the rest of the ingredients in a bowl, toss and serve cold.

Nutrition:

160 Calories 4.3g Fat 10g Protein

14g Carbohydrates

5.   Cranberry Bulgur Mix

Difficulty: Novice level

Preparation Time: 10 minutes

Cooking Time: 0 minutes

Servings: 4

Size/ Portion: 2 cups

Ingredients:

- 1 and ½ cups hot water
- 1 cup bulgur
- Juice of ½ lemon
- 4 tablespoons cilantro, chopped
- ½ cup cranberries
- 1 and ½ teaspoons curry powder
- ¼ cup green onions
- ½ cup red bell peppers
- ½ cup carrots, grated
- 1 tablespoon olive oil

Directions:

1. Put bulgur into a bowl, add the water, stir, cover, leave aside for 10 minutes, fluff with a fork, and transfer to a bowl. Add the rest of the ingredients, toss, and serve cold.

Nutrition:

300 Calories 6.4g Fat

13g Protein 18g Carbohydrates

6.   Chickpeas, Corn and Black Beans Salad

Difficulty: Novice level

Preparation Time: 10 minutes

Cooking Time: 0 minutes

Servings: 4

Size/ Portion: 2 cups

Ingredients:

- 1 and ½ cups canned black beans
- ½ teaspoon garlic powder
- 2 teaspoons chili powder
- 1 and ½ cups canned chickpeas
- 1 cup baby spinach
- 1 avocado, pitted, peeled, and chopped
- 1 cup corn kernels, chopped
- 2 tablespoons lemon juice
- 1 tablespoon olive oil
- 1 tablespoon apple cider vinegar
- 1 teaspoon chives, chopped

Directions:

1. Mix the black beans with the garlic powder, chili powder, and the rest of the ingredients in a bowl, toss and serve cold.

Nutrition:

300 Calories

13.4g Fat

13g Protein

16g Carbohydrates

7.   Olives and Lentils Salad

Difficulty: Novice level

Preparation Time: 10 minutes

Cooking Time: 0 minutes

Servings: 2

Size/ Portion: 2 cups

Ingredients:

- 1/3 cup canned green lentils
- 1 tablespoon olive oil
- 2 cups baby spinach
- 1 cup black olives
- 2 tablespoons sunflower seeds
- 1 tablespoon Dijon mustard
- 2 tablespoons balsamic vinegar
- 2 tablespoons olive oil

Directions:

1. Mix the lentils with the spinach, olives, and the rest of the ingredients in a salad bowl, toss and serve cold.

Nutrition:

279 Calories 6.5g Fat

12g Protein 13g Carbohydrates

8. Lime Spinach and Chickpeas Salad

Difficulty: Novice level

Preparation Time: 10 minutes

Cooking Time: 0 minutes

Servings: 4

Size/ Portion: 2 cups

Ingredients:

- 16 ounces canned chickpeas
- 2 cups baby spinach leaves
- ½ tablespoon lime juice
- 2 tablespoons olive oil
- 1 teaspoon cumin, ground
- ½ teaspoon chili flakes

Directions:

1. Mix the chickpeas with the spinach and the rest of the ingredients in a large bowl, toss and serve cold.

Nutrition: 240 calories 8.2g fat

12g protein 7.9g Carbohydrates

9. Minty Olives and Tomatoes Salad

Difficulty: Novice level

Preparation Time: 10 minutes

Cooking Time: 0 minutes

Servings: 4

Size/ Portion: 2 cups

Ingredients:

- 1 cup kalamata olives
- 1 cup black olives
- 1 cup cherry tomatoes
- 4 tomatoes
- 1 red onion, chopped
- 2 tablespoons oregano, chopped
- 1 tablespoon mint, chopped
- 2 tablespoons balsamic vinegar
- ¼ cup olive oil
- 2 teaspoons Italian herbs, dried

Directions:

1. In a salad bowl, mix the olives with the tomatoes and the rest of the ingredients, toss, and serve cold.

Nutrition: 190 Calories 8.1g Fat

4.6g Protein 5.7g Carbohydrates

10. Beans and Cucumber Salad

Difficulty: Novice level

Preparation Time: 10 minutes

Cooking Time: 0 minutes

Servings: 4

Size/ Portion: 2 cups

Ingredients:

- 15 g canned great northern beans
- 2 tablespoons olive oil
- ½ cup baby arugula
- 1 cup cucumber
- 1 tablespoon parsley
- 2 tomatoes, cubed
- 2 tablespoon balsamic vinegar

Directions:

1. Mix the beans with the cucumber and the rest of the ingredients in a large bowl, toss and serve cold.

Nutrition: 233 calories 9g fat

8g protein 9g Carbohydrates

11. Tomato and Avocado Salad

Difficulty: Intermediate level

Preparation Time: 10 minutes

Cooking Time: 0 minutes

Servings: 4

Size/ Portion: 2 cups

Ingredients:

- 1-pound cherry tomatoes
- 2 avocados
- 1 sweet onion, chopped
- 2 tablespoons lemon juice
- 1 and ½ tablespoons olive oil
- Handful basil, chopped

Directions:

1. Mix the tomatoes with the avocados and the rest of the ingredients in a serving bowl, toss and serve right away.

Nutrition:

148 Calories 7.8g Fat

5.5g Protein 8.1g Carbohydrates

12. Arugula Salad

Difficulty: Novice level

Preparation Time: 5 minutes

Cooking Time: 0 minutes

Servings: 4

Size/ Portion: 2 cups

Ingredients:

- Arugula leaves (4 cups)
- Cherry tomatoes (1 cup)
- Pine nuts (.25 cup)
- Rice vinegar (1 tbsp.)
- Olive/grapeseed oil (2 tbsp.)
- Grated parmesan cheese (.25 cup)
- Black pepper & salt (as desired)
- Large sliced avocado (1)

Directions:

1. Peel and slice the avocado. Rinse and dry the arugula leaves, grate the cheese, and slice the cherry tomatoes into halves.
2. Combine the arugula, pine nuts, tomatoes, oil, vinegar, salt, pepper, and cheese.
3. Toss the salad to mix and portion it onto plates with the avocado slices to serve.

Nutrition:

257 Calories

23g Fats

6.1g Protein

12g Carbohydrates

13. Chickpea Salad

Difficulty: Novice level

Preparation Time: 15 minutes

Cooking Time: 0 minutes

Servings: 4

Size/ Portion: 2 cups

Ingredients:

- Cooked chickpeas (15 g)
- Diced Roma tomato (1)
- Diced green medium bell pepper (half of 1)
- Fresh parsley (1 tbsp.)
- Small white onion (1)
- Minced garlic (.5 tsp.)
- Lemon (1 juiced)

Directions:

1. Chop the tomato, green pepper, and onion. Mince the garlic. Combine each of the fixings into a salad bowl and toss well.
2. Cover the salad to chill for at least 15 minutes in the fridge. Serve when ready.

Nutrition: 163 Calories 7g Fats

4g Protein 5g Carbohydrates

- 2 cups of water
- 1 1/2 teaspoons oregano
- 1/2 teaspoon basil
- 1/4 teaspoon thyme
- 1 teaspoon salt
- 1/2 teaspoon pepper
- 3/4 cup small pasta shells
- 4 cups fresh baby spinach
- 1/4 cup Parmesan or Romano cheese

Direction:

1. Grab a stockpot and place over medium heat. Add the oil then the onions, garlic, carrots, zucchini, squash, parsley, and celery. Cook for five minutes until the veggies are getting soft.

2. Pour in the stock, water, beans, tomatoes, herbs, and salt and pepper. Stir well. Decrease heat, cover, and simmer for 30 minutes.

3. Add the pasta and spinach, stir well then cover and cook for a further 20 minutes until the pasta is cooked through. Stir through the cheese then serve and enjoy.

Nutrition:

34 calories

26.3 g protein

30.3 g fat

28.7g Carbohydrates

2. Chicken Wild Rice Soup

Difficulty: Novice level

Preparation Time: 10 minutes

Cooking Time: 15 minutes

Servings: 6

Size/ Portion: 1 cup

Ingredients:

- 2/3 cup wild rice, uncooked
- 1 tablespoon onion, chopped finely

- 1 tablespoon fresh parsley, chopped
- 1 cup carrots, chopped
- 8-ounces chicken breast, cooked
- 2 tablespoon butter
- 1/4 cup all-purpose white flour
- 5 cups low-sodium chicken broth
- 1 tablespoon slivered almonds

Directions:

1. Start by adding rice and 2 cups broth along with ½ cup water to a cooking pot. Cook the chicken until the rice is al dente and set it aside. Add butter to a saucepan and melt it.

2. Stir in onion and sauté until soft then add the flour and the remaining broth.

3. Stir it and then cook for it 1 minute then add the chicken, cooked rice, and carrots. Cook for 5 minutes on simmer. Garnish with almonds. Serve fresh.

Nutrition:

287 calories 21g protein

35g fat 31g Carbohydrates

3. Classic Chicken Soup

Difficulty: Novice level

Preparation Time: 10 minutes

Cooking Time: 25 minutes

Servings: 2

Size/ Portion: 1 cup

Ingredients:

- 1 1/2 cups low-sodium vegetable broth
- 1 cup of water
- 1/4 teaspoon poultry seasoning
- 1/4 teaspoon black pepper
- 1 cup chicken strips
- 1/4 cup carrot
- 2-ounces egg noodles, uncooked

11.   Tomato and Avocado Salad

Difficulty: Intermediate level

Preparation Time: 10 minutes

Cooking Time: 0 minutes

Servings: 4

Size/ Portion: 2 cups

Ingredients:

- 1-pound cherry tomatoes
- 2 avocados
- 1 sweet onion, chopped
- 2 tablespoons lemon juice
- 1 and ½ tablespoons olive oil
- Handful basil, chopped

Directions:

1. Mix the tomatoes with the avocados and the rest of the ingredients in a serving bowl, toss and serve right away.

Nutrition:

148 Calories 7.8g Fat

5.5g Protein 8.1g Carbohydrates

12.   Arugula Salad

Difficulty: Novice level

Preparation Time: 5 minutes

Cooking Time: 0 minutes

Servings: 4

Size/ Portion: 2 cups

Ingredients:

- Arugula leaves (4 cups)
- Cherry tomatoes (1 cup)
- Pine nuts (.25 cup)
- Rice vinegar (1 tbsp.)
- Olive/grapeseed oil (2 tbsp.)
- Grated parmesan cheese (.25 cup)
- Black pepper & salt (as desired)
- Large sliced avocado (1)

Directions:

1. Peel and slice the avocado. Rinse and dry the arugula leaves, grate the cheese, and slice the cherry tomatoes into halves.
2. Combine the arugula, pine nuts, tomatoes, oil, vinegar, salt, pepper, and cheese.
3. Toss the salad to mix and portion it onto plates with the avocado slices to serve.

Nutrition:

257 Calories

23g Fats

6.1g Protein

12g Carbohydrates

13.   Chickpea Salad

Difficulty: Novice level

Preparation Time: 15 minutes

Cooking Time: 0 minutes

Servings: 4

Size/ Portion: 2 cups

Ingredients:

- Cooked chickpeas (15 g)
- Diced Roma tomato (1)
- Diced green medium bell pepper (half of 1)
- Fresh parsley (1 tbsp.)
- Small white onion (1)
- Minced garlic (.5 tsp.)
- Lemon (1 juiced)

Directions:

1. Chop the tomato, green pepper, and onion. Mince the garlic. Combine each of the fixings into a salad bowl and toss well.
2. Cover the salad to chill for at least 15 minutes in the fridge. Serve when ready.

Nutrition: 163 Calories 7g Fats

4g Protein 5g Carbohydrates

14. Chopped Israeli Mediterranean Pasta Salad

Difficulty: Novice level

Preparation Time: 15 minutes

Cooking Time: 2 minutes

Servings: 8

Size/ Portion: 2 cups

Ingredients:

- Small bow tie or other small pasta (.5 lb.)
- 1/3 cup Cucumber
- 1/3 cup Radish
- 1/3 cup Tomato
- 1/3 cup Yellow bell pepper
- 1/3 cup Orange bell pepper
- 1/3 cup Black olives
- 1/3 cup Green olives
- 1/3 cup Red onions
- 1/3 cup Pepperoncini
- 1/3 cup Feta cheese
- 1/3 cup Fresh thyme leaves
- Dried oregano (1 tsp.)

Dressing:

- 0.25 cup + more, olive oil
- juice of 1 lemon

Directions:

1. Slice the green olives into halves. Dice the feta and pepperoncini. Finely dice the remainder of the veggies.
2. Prepare a pot of water with the salt, and simmer the pasta until its al dente (checking at two minutes under the listed time). Rinse and drain in cold water.
3. Combine a small amount of oil with the pasta. Add the salt, pepper, oregano, thyme, and veggies. Pour in the rest of the oil, lemon juice, and mix and fold in the grated feta.

4. Pop it into the fridge within two hours, best if overnight. Taste test and adjust the seasonings to your liking; add fresh thyme.

Nutrition:

65 Calories

5.6g Fats

0.8g Protein

6.9g Carbohydrates

15. Feta Tomato Salad

Difficulty: Novice level

Preparation Time: 5 minutes

Cooking Time: 0 minutes

Servings: 4

Size/ Portion: 2 cups

Ingredients:

- Balsamic vinegar (2 tbsp.)
- Freshly minced basil (1.5 tsp.) or dried (.5 tsp.)
- Salt (.5 tsp.)
- Coarsely chopped sweet onion (.5 cup)
- Olive oil (2 tbsp.)
- Cherry or grape tomatoes (1 lb.)
- Crumbled feta cheese (.25 cup.)

Directions:

1. Whisk the salt, basil, and vinegar. Toss the onion into the vinegar mixture for 5 minutes
2. Slice the tomatoes into halves and stir in the tomatoes, feta cheese, and oil to serve.

Nutrition:

121 Calories

9g Fats

3g Protein

8g Carbohydrates

16.   Greek Pasta Salad

Difficulty: Novice level

Preparation Time: 5 minutes

Cooking Time: 11 minutes

Servings: 4

Size/ Portion: 2 cups

Ingredients:

- Penne pasta (1 cup)
- Lemon juice (1.5 tsp.)
- Red wine vinegar (2 tbsp.)
- Garlic (1 clove)
- Dried oregano (1 tsp.)
- Black pepper and sea salt (as desired)
- Olive oil (.33 cup)
- Halved cherry tomatoes (5)
- Red onion (half of 1 small)
- Green & red bell pepper (half of 1 - each) - Cucumber (¼ of 1)
- Black olives (.25 cup)
- Crumbled feta cheese (.25 cup)

Directions:

1. Slice the cucumber and olives. Chop/dice the onion, peppers, and garlic. Slice the tomatoes into halves.

2. Arrange a large pot with water and salt using the high-temperature setting. Once it's boiling, add the pasta and cook for 11 minutes Rinse it using cold water and drain in a colander.

3. Whisk the oil, juice, salt, pepper, vinegar, oregano, and garlic. Combine the cucumber, cheese, olives, peppers, pasta, onions, and tomatoes in a large salad dish.

4. Add the vinaigrette over the pasta and toss. Chill in the fridge (covered) for about three hours and serve as desired.

Nutrition:

307 Calories 23.6g Fat 5.4g Protein

3.8g Carbohydrates

Lunch and Dinner (Soup and Stew)

1.   Minestrone Soup

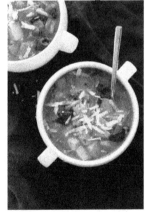

Difficulty: Novice level

Preparation Time: 10 minutes

Cooking Time: 1 hour

Servings: 4

Size/ Portion: 1 cup

Ingredients:

- 1 small white onion
- 4 cloves garlic
- 1/2 cup carrots
- 1 medium zucchini
- 1 medium yellow squash
- 2 tablespoons minced fresh parsley
- 1/4 cup celery sliced
- 3 tablespoons olive oil
- 2 x 15 g cans cannellini beans
- 2 x 15 g can red kidney beans
- 1 x 14.5 g can fire-roasted diced tomatoes, drained
- 4 cups vegetable stock

- 2 cups of water
- 1 1/2 teaspoons oregano
- 1/2 teaspoon basil
- 1/4 teaspoon thyme
- 1 teaspoon salt
- 1/2 teaspoon pepper
- 3/4 cup small pasta shells
- 4 cups fresh baby spinach
- 1/4 cup Parmesan or Romano cheese

Direction:

1. Grab a stockpot and place over medium heat. Add the oil then the onions, garlic, carrots, zucchini, squash, parsley, and celery. Cook for five minutes until the veggies are getting soft.

2. Pour in the stock, water, beans, tomatoes, herbs, and salt and pepper. Stir well. Decrease heat, cover, and simmer for 30 minutes.

3. Add the pasta and spinach, stir well then cover and cook for a further 20 minutes until the pasta is cooked through. Stir through the cheese then serve and enjoy.

Nutrition:

34 calories

26.3 g protein

30.3 g fat

28.7g Carbohydrates

2.   Chicken Wild Rice Soup

Difficulty: Novice level

Preparation Time: 10 minutes

Cooking Time: 15 minutes

Servings: 6

Size/ Portion: 1 cup

Ingredients:

- 2/3 cup wild rice, uncooked
- 1 tablespoon onion, chopped finely

- 1 tablespoon fresh parsley, chopped
- 1 cup carrots, chopped
- 8-ounces chicken breast, cooked
- 2 tablespoon butter
- 1/4 cup all-purpose white flour
- 5 cups low-sodium chicken broth
- 1 tablespoon slivered almonds

Directions:

1. Start by adding rice and 2 cups broth along with ½ cup water to a cooking pot. Cook the chicken until the rice is al dente and set it aside. Add butter to a saucepan and melt it.

2. Stir in onion and sauté until soft then add the flour and the remaining broth.

3. Stir it and then cook for it 1 minute then add the chicken, cooked rice, and carrots. Cook for 5 minutes on simmer. Garnish with almonds. Serve fresh.

Nutrition:

287 calories 21g protein

35g fat 31g Carbohydrates

3.   Classic Chicken Soup

Difficulty: Novice level

Preparation Time: 10 minutes

Cooking Time: 25 minutes

Servings: 2

Size/ Portion: 1 cup

Ingredients:

- 1 1/2 cups low-sodium vegetable broth
- 1 cup of water
- 1/4 teaspoon poultry seasoning
- 1/4 teaspoon black pepper
- 1 cup chicken strips
- 1/4 cup carrot
- 2-ounces egg noodles, uncooked

Directions:

1. Gather all the ingredients into a slow cooker and toss it Cook soup on high heat for 25 minutes.

2. Serve warm.

Nutrition:

103 calories

8g protein

11g fat

11g Carbohydrates

4. Cucumber Soup

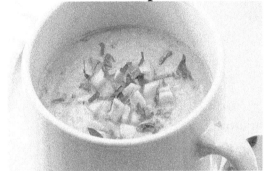

Difficulty: Novice level

Preparation Time: 10 minutes

Cooking Time: 0 minute

Servings: 4

Size/ Portion: 1 cup

Ingredients:

- 2 medium cucumbers
- 1/3 cup sweet white onion
- 1 green onion
- 1/4 cup fresh mint
- 2 tablespoons fresh dill
- 2 tablespoons lemon juice
- 2/3 cup water
- 1/2 cup half and half cream
- 1/3 cup sour cream
- 1/2 teaspoon pepper
- Fresh dill sprigs for garnish

Directions:

1. Situate all of the ingredients into a food processor and toss. Puree the mixture and refrigerate for 2 hours. Garnish with dill sprigs. Enjoy fresh.

Nutrition:

77 calories

2g protein

6g fats

5g Carbohydrates

5. Squash and Turmeric Soup

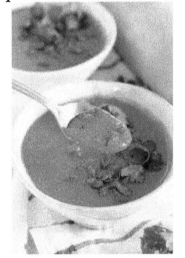

Difficulty: Novice level

Preparation Time: 10 minutes

Cooking Time: 30 minutes

Servings: 4

Size/ Portion: 1 cup

Ingredients:

- 4 cups low-sodium vegetable broth
- 2 medium zucchini squash
- 2 medium yellow crookneck squash
- 1 small onion
- 1/2 cup frozen green peas
- 2 tablespoons olive oil
- 1/2 cup plain nonfat Greek yogurt
- 2 teaspoon turmeric

Directions:

1. Warm the broth in a saucepan on medium heat. Toss in onion, squash, and zucchini. Let it simmer for approximately 25 minutes then add oil and green peas.

2. Cook for another 5 minutes then allow it to cool. Puree the soup using a handheld blender then add Greek yogurt and turmeric. Refrigerate it overnight and serve fresh.

Nutrition:

100 calories 4g protein

10g fat 12g Carbohydrates

6. Leek, Potato, and Carrot Soup

Difficulty: Novice level

Preparation Time: 15 minutes

Cooking Time: 25 minutes

Servings: 4

Size/ Portion: 1 cup

Ingredients:

- 1 - leek
- ¾ - cup diced and boiled potatoes
- ¾ - cup diced and boiled carrots
- 1 - garlic clove
- 1 - tablespoon oil
- Crushed pepper to taste
- 3 - cups low sodium chicken stock
- Chopped parsley for garnish
- 1 - bay leaf
- ¼ - teaspoon ground cumin

Directions:

1. Trim off and take away a portion of the coarse inexperienced portions of the leek, at that factor reduce daintily and flush altogether in virus water. Channel properly. Warmth the oil in an extensively based pot. Include the leek

and garlic, and sear over low warmth for two-3 minutes, till sensitive.

2. Include the inventory, inlet leaf, cumin, and pepper. Heat the mixture, mix constantly. Include the bubbled potatoes and carrots and stew for 10-15minutes Modify the flavoring, eliminate the inlet leaf, and serve sprinkled generously with slashed parsley.

3. To make a pureed soup, manner the soup in a blender or nourishment processor till smooth Come again to the pan. Include ½ field milk. Bring to bubble and stew for 2-3minutes

Nutrition:

315 calories 8g fat

15g protein 7g Carbohydrates

7. Bell Pepper Soup

Difficulty: Novice level

Preparation Time: 30 minutes

Cooking Time: 35 minutes

Servings: 4

Size/ Portion: 1 cup

Ingredients:

- 4 - cups low-sodium chicken broth
- 3 - red peppers
- 2 - medium onions
- 3 - tablespoon lemon juice
- 1 - tablespoon finely minced lemon zest
- A pinch cayenne peppers
- ¼ - teaspoon cinnamon
- ½ - cup finely minced fresh cilantro

Directions:

1. In a medium stockpot, consolidate each one of the fixings except for the cilantro and warmth to the point of boiling over excessive warm temperature.

2. Diminish the warmth and stew, ordinarily secured, for around 30

minutes, till thickened. Cool marginally. Utilizing a hand blender or nourishment processor, puree the soup. Include the cilantro and tenderly heat.

Nutrition:

265 calories 8g fat

5g protein 7g Carbohydrates

8.   Yucatan Soup

Difficulty: Novice level

Preparation Time: 10 minutes

Cooking Time: 20 minutes

Servings: 4

Size/ Portion: 1 cup

Ingredients:

- ½ cup onion, chopped
- 8 cloves garlic, chopped
- 2 Serrano chili peppers, chopped
- 1 medium tomato, chopped
- 1 ½ cups chicken breast, cooked, shredded
- 2 six-inch corn tortillas, sliced
- 1 tablespoon olive oil
- 4 cups chicken broth
- 1 bay leaf
- ¼ cup lime juice
- ¼ cup cilantro, chopped
- 1 teaspoon black pepper

Directions:

1. Spread the corn tortillas in a baking sheet and bake them for 3 minutes at 400°F. Place a suitably-sized saucepan over medium heat and add oil to heat.

2. Toss in chili peppers, garlic, and onion, then sauté until soft. Stir in broth, tomatoes, bay leaf, and chicken.

3. Let this chicken soup cook for 10 minutes on a simmer. Stir in cilantro, lime juice, and black pepper. Garnish with baked corn tortillas. Serve.

Nutrition:

215 calories 21g protein 32g fat

28g Carbohydrates

9.   Zesty Taco Soup

Difficulty: Novice level

Preparation Time: 10 minutes

Cooking Time: 7 hours

Servings: 2

Size/ Portion: 1 cup

Ingredients:

- 1 ½ pounds chicken breast
- 15 ½ ounces canned dark red kidney beans
- 15 ½ ounces canned white corn
- 1 cup canned tomatoes
- ½ cup onion
- 15 ½ ounces canned yellow hominy
- ½ cup green bell peppers
- 1 garlic clove
- 1 medium jalapeno
- 1 tablespoon package McCormick
- 2 cups chicken broth

Directions:

1. Add drained beans, hominy, corn, onion, garlic, jalapeno pepper, chicken, and green peppers to a Crockpot.

2. Cover the beans-corn mixture and cook for 1 hour on "high" temperature. Set heat to "low" and continue cooking for 6 hours. Shred the slow-cooked chicken and return to the taco soup. Serve warm.

Nutrition:

191 calories 21g protein

20g fat17g Carbohydrates

10. Southwestern Posole

Difficulty: Intermediate level

Preparation Time: 10 minutes

Cooking Time: 53 minutes

Servings: 4

Size/ Portion: 1 cup

Ingredients:

- 1 tablespoon olive oil
- 1-pound pork loin, diced
- ½ cup onion, chopped
- 1 garlic clove, chopped
- 28 ounces canned white hominy
- 4 ounces canned diced green chilis
- 4 cups chicken broth
- ¼ teaspoon black pepper

Directions:

1. Place a suitably-sized cooking pot over medium heat and add oil to heat. Toss in pork pieces and sauté for 4 minutes.
2. Stir in garlic and onion, then stir for 4 minutes, or until onion is soft. Add the remaining ingredients, then cover the pork soup. Cook this for 45 minutes, or until the pork is tender. Serve warm.

Nutrition:

286 calories 25g protein 15g fat

28g Carbohydrates

11. Spring Vegetable Soup

Difficulty: Intermediate level

Preparation Time: 10 minutes

Cooking Time: 45 minutes

Servings: 4

Size/ Portion: 1 cup

Ingredients:

- 1 cup fresh green beans
- ¾ cup celery

- ½ cup onion
- ½ cup carrots
- ½ cup mushrooms
- ½ cup of frozen corn
- 1 medium Roma tomato
- 2 tablespoons olive oil
- ½ cup of frozen corn
- 4 cups vegetable broth
- 1 teaspoon dried oregano leaves
- 1 teaspoon garlic powder

Directions:

1. Place a suitably-sized cooking pot over medium heat and add olive oil to heat. Toss in onion and celery, then sauté until soft. Stir in the corn and rest of the ingredients and cook the soup to boil.
2. Now reduce its heat to a simmer and cook for 45 minutes. Serve warm.

Nutrition:115 calories 3g protein 13g fat

16g Carbohydrates

12. Seafood Corn Chowder

Difficulty: Intermediate level

Preparation Time: 10 minutes

Cooking Time: 12 minutes

Servings: 4

Size/ Portion: 1 cup

Ingredients:

- 1 tablespoon butter
- 1 cup onion
- 1/3 cup celery
- ½ cup green bell pepper
- ½ cup red bell pepper
- 1 tablespoon white flour
- 14 ounces chicken broth
- 2 cups cream

- 6 ounces evaporated milk
- 10 ounces surimi imitation crab chunks
- 2 cups frozen corn kernels
- ½ teaspoon black pepper
- ½ teaspoon paprika

Directions:

1. Place a suitably-sized saucepan over medium heat and add butter to melt. Toss in onion, green and red peppers, and celery, then sauté for 5 minutes. Stir in flour and whisk well for 2 minutes.
2. Pour in chicken broth and stir until it boils. Add evaporated milk, corn, surimi crab, paprika, black pepper, and creamer. Cook for 5 minutes then serves warm.

Nutrition:

175 calories

8g protein

7g fat

9g Carbohydrates

13. Beef Sage Soup
Difficulty: Intermediate level

Preparation Time: 10 minutes

Cooking Time: 20 minutes

Servings: 4

Size/ Portion: 1 cup

Ingredients:

- ½ pound ground beef
- ½ teaspoon ground sage
- ½ teaspoon black pepper
- ½ teaspoon dried basil
- ½ teaspoon garlic powder
- 4 slices bread, cubed
- 2 tablespoons olive oil
- 1 tablespoon herb seasoning blend
- 2 garlic cloves, minced

- 3 cups chicken broth
- 1 ½ cups water
- 4 tablespoons fresh parsley
- 2 tablespoons parmesan cheese

Directions:

1. Preheat your oven to 375°F. Mix beef with sage, basil, black pepper, and garlic powder in a bowl, then set it aside. Toss the bread cubes with olive oil in a baking sheet and bake them for 8 minutes.
2. Meanwhile, sauté the beef mixture in a greased cooking pot until it is browned. Stir in garlic and sauté for 2 minutes, then add parsley, water, and broth. Cover the beef soup and cook for 10 minutes on a simmer. Garnish the soup with parmesan cheese and baked bread. Serve warm.

Nutrition:

336 calories

26g protein

16g fat

23g Carbohydrates

14. Cabbage Borscht
Difficulty: Intermediate level

Preparation Time: 10 minutes

Cooking Time: 90 minutes

Servings: 6

Size/ Portion: 1 cup

Ingredients:

- 2 pounds beef steaks
- 6 cups cold water
- 2 tablespoons olive oil
- ½ cup tomato sauce
- 1 medium cabbage, chopped
- 1 cup onion, diced
- 1 cup carrots, diced

- 1 cup turnips, peeled and diced
- 1 teaspoon pepper
- 6 tablespoons lemon juice
- 4 tablespoons sugar

Directions:

1. Start by placing steak in a large cooking pot and pour enough water to cover it. Cover the beef pot and cook it on a simmer until it is tender, then shred it using a fork. Add olive oil, onion, tomato sauce, carrots, turnips, and shredded steak to the cooking liquid in the pot.

2. Stir in black pepper, sugar, and lemon juice to season the soup. Cover the cabbage soup and cook on low heat for 1 ½ hour. Serve warm.

Nutrition:

212 calories

19g protein

10g fat

17g Carbohydrates

CHAPTER 9:

Fruits and Dessert Recipes

1.   Chocolate Ganache

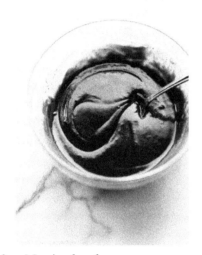

Difficulty: Novice level

Preparation Time: 10 minutes

Cooking Time: 16 minutes

Servings: 16

Size/ Portion: 2 tablespoons

Ingredients

- 9 ounces bittersweet chocolate, chopped
- 1 cup heavy cream
- 1 tablespoon dark rum (optional)

Direction

1. Situate chocolate in a medium bowl. Cook cream in a small saucepan over medium heat.
2. Bring to a boil. When the cream has reached a boiling point, pour the chopped chocolate over it and beat until smooth. Stir the rum if desired.

3. Allow the ganache to cool slightly before you pour it on a cake. Begin in the middle of the cake and work outside. For a fluffy icing or chocolate filling, let it cool until thick and beat with a whisk until light and fluffy.

Nutrition:

142 calories 10.8g fat 1.4g protein

2.   Chocolate Covered Strawberries

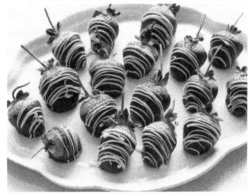

Difficulty: Novice level

Preparation Time: 15 minutes

Cooking Time: 0 minute

Servings: 24

Size/ Portion: 2 pieces

Ingredients

- 16 ounces milk chocolate chips
- 2 tablespoons shortening
- 1-pound fresh strawberries with leaves

Direction

1. In a bain-marie, melt chocolate and shortening, occasionally stirring until smooth. Pierce the tops of the

strawberries with toothpicks and immerse them in the chocolate mixture.

2. Turn the strawberries and put the toothpick in Styrofoam so that the chocolate cools.

Nutrition: 115 calories 7.3g fat 1.4g protein 24g Carbohydrates

3. Strawberry Angel Food Dessert

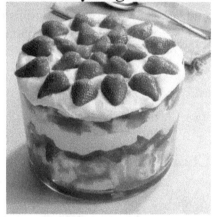

Difficulty: Novice level

Preparation Time: 15 minutes

Cooking Time: 0 minutes

Servings: 18

Size/ Portion: 1 cup

Ingredients

- 1 angel cake (10 inches)
- 2 packages of softened cream cheese
- 1 cup of white sugar
- 1 container (8 g) of frozen fluff, thawed
- 1 liter of fresh strawberries, sliced
- 1 jar of strawberry icing

Direction

1. Crumble the cake in a 9 x 13-inch dish.
2. Beat the cream cheese and sugar in a medium bowl until the mixture is light and fluffy. Stir in the whipped topping. Crush the cake with your hands, and spread the cream cheese mixture over the cake.

3. Combine the strawberries and the frosting in a bowl until the strawberries are well covered. Spread over the layer of cream cheese. Cool until ready to serve.

Nutrition: 261 calories 11g fat 3.2g protein 17g Carbohydrates

4. Fruit Pizza

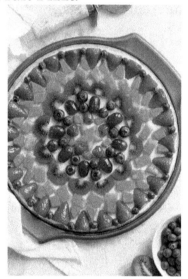

Difficulty: Novice level

Preparation Time: 30 minutes

Cooking Time: 0 minute

Servings: 8

Size/ Portion: 1 slice

Ingredients

- 1 (18-oz) package sugar cookie dough
- 1 (8-oz) package cream cheese, softened
- 1 (8-oz) frozen filling, defrosted
- 2 cups of freshly cut strawberries
- 1/2 cup of white sugar
- 1 pinch of salt
- 1 tablespoon corn flour
- 2 tablespoons lemon juice
- 1/2 cup orange juice
- 1/4 cup water
- 1/2 teaspoon orange zest

Direction

1. Ready oven to 175 ° C Slice the cookie dough then place it on a greased pizza pan. Press the dough flat into the mold. Bake for 10 to 12 minutes. Let cool.

2. Soften the cream cheese in a large bowl and then stir in the whipped topping. Spread over the cooled crust.

3. Start with strawberries cut in half. Situate in a circle around the outer edge. Continue with the fruit of your choice by going to the center. If you use bananas, immerse them in lemon juice. Then make a sauce with a spoon on the fruit.

4. Combine sugar, salt, corn flour, orange juice, lemon juice, and water in a pan. Boil and stir over medium heat. Boil for 1 or 2 minutes until thick. Remove from heat and add the grated orange zest. Place on the fruit.

5. Allow to cool for two hours, cut into quarters, and serve.

Nutrition 535 calories 30g fat

5.5g protein 14g Carbohydrates

5. Rhubarb Strawberry Crunch

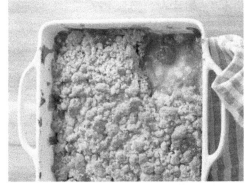

Difficulty: Novice level

Preparation Time: 15 minutes

Cooking Time: 45 minutes

Servings: 18

Size/ Portion: 1 cup

Ingredients

- 1 cup of white sugar

- 3 tablespoons all-purpose flour

- 3 cups of fresh strawberries, sliced

- 3 cups of rhubarb, cut into cubes

- 1 1/2 cup flour

- 1 cup packed brown sugar

- 1 cup butter

- 1 cup oatmeal

Direction

1. Preheat the oven to 190 ° C.

2. Combine white sugar, 3 tablespoons flour, strawberries and rhubarb in a large bowl. Place the mixture in a 9 x 13-inch baking dish.

3. Mix 1 1/2 cups of flour, brown sugar, butter, and oats until a crumbly texture is obtained. You may want to use a blender for this. Crumble the mixture of rhubarb and strawberry.

4. Bake for 45 minutes.

Nutrition:

253 calories 10.8g fat

2.3g protein 7.8g Carbohydrates

6. Chocolate Chip Banana Dessert

Difficulty: Novice level

Preparation Time: 20 minutes

Cooking Time: 20 minutes

Servings: 24

Size/ Portion:

Ingredients

- 2/3 cup white sugar

- 3/4 cup butter

- 2/3 cup brown sugar

- 1 egg, beaten slightly

- 1 teaspoon vanilla extract

- 1 cup of banana puree

- 1 3/4 cup flour

- 2 teaspoons baking powder
- 1/2 teaspoon of salt
- 1 cup of semi-sweet chocolate chips

Direction:

1. Ready the oven to 175 ° C Grease and bake a 10 x 15-inch baking pan.

2. Beat the butter, white sugar, and brown sugar in a large bowl until light. Beat the egg and vanilla. Fold in the banana puree: mix baking powder, flour, and salt in another bowl. Mix flour mixture into the butter mixture. Stir in the chocolate chips. Spread in pan.

3. Bake for 20 minutes. Cool before cutting into squares.

Nutrition:

174 calories

8.2g fat

1.7g protein

8.7g Carbohydrates

7. Apple Pie Filling

Difficulty: Novice level

Preparation Time: 20 minutes

Cooking Time: 12 minutes

Servings: 40

Size/ Portion: 1 cup

Ingredients

- 18 cups chopped apples
- 3 tablespoons lemon juice
- 10 cups of water
- 4 1/2 cups of white sugar
- 1 cup corn flour
- 2 teaspoons of ground cinnamon
- 1 teaspoon of salt
- 1/4 teaspoon ground nutmeg

Direction

1. Mix apples with lemon juice in a large bowl and set aside. Pour the water in a Dutch oven over medium heat. Combine sugar, corn flour, cinnamon, salt, and nutmeg in a bowl. Add to water, mix well, and bring to a boil. Cook for 2 minutes with continuous stirring.

2. Boil apples again. Reduce the heat, cover, and simmer for 8 minutes. Allow cooling for 30 minutes.

3. Pour into five freezer containers and leave 1/2 inch of free space. Cool to room temperature.

4. Seal and freeze

Nutrition:

129 calories

0.1g fat

0.2g protein

1.9g Carbohydrates

8. Ice Cream Sandwich Dessert

Difficulty: Novice level

Preparation Time: 20 minutes

Cooking Time: 0 minute

Servings: 12

Size/ Portion: 2 squares

Ingredients

- 22 ice cream sandwiches
- Frozen whipped topping in 16 g container, thawed
- 1 jar (12 g) Caramel ice cream
- 1 1/2 cups of salted peanuts

Direction

1. Cut a sandwich with ice in two. Place a whole sandwich and a half sandwich on a short side of a 9 x 13-inch baking dish. Repeat this until the bottom is covered, alternate the full sandwich, and the half sandwich.

2. Spread half of the whipped topping. Pour the caramel over it. Sprinkle with half the peanuts. Do layers with the rest of the ice cream sandwiches, whipped cream, and peanuts.

3. Cover and freeze for up to 2 months. Remove from the freezer 20 minutes before serving. Cut into squares.

Nutrition:

559 calories

28.8g fat

10g protein

13g Carbohydrates

9.   Cranberry and Pistachio Biscotti

Difficulty: Novice level

Preparation Time: 15 minutes

Cooking Time: 35 minutes

Servings: 36

Size/ Portion: 2 slices

Ingredients

- 1/4 cup light olive oil
- 3/4 cup white sugar
- 2 teaspoons vanilla extract
- 1/2 teaspoon almond extract
- 2 eggs
- 1 3/4 cup all-purpose flour
- 1/4 teaspoon salt
- 1 teaspoon baking powder
- 1/2 cup dried cranberries
- 1 1/2 cup pistachio nuts

Direction

1. Prep oven to 150 ° C

2. Combine the oil and sugar in a large bowl until a homogeneous mixture is obtained. Stir in the vanilla and almond extract and add the eggs. Combine flour, salt, and baking powder; gradually add to

the egg mixture — mix cranberries and nuts by hand.

3. Divide the dough in half — form two 12 x 2-inch logs on a parchment baking sheet. The dough can be sticky, wet hands with cold water to make it easier to handle the dough.

4. Bake in the preheated oven for 35 minutes or until the blocks are golden brown. Pullout from the oven and let cool for 10 minutes. Reduce oven heat to 275 degrees F (135 degrees C).

5. Cut diagonally into 3/4-inch-thick slices. Place on the sides on the baking sheet covered with parchment — Bake for about 8 to 10 minutes

Nutrition:

92 calories

4.3g fat

2.1g protein

11g Carbohydrates

10.   Cream Puff Dessert

Difficulty: Novice level

Preparation Time: 20 minutes

Cooking Time: 36 minutes

Servings: 12

Size/ Portion: 2 puffs

Ingredients

Puff

- 1 cup water
- 1/2 cup butter
- 1 cup all-purpose flour
- 4 eggs

Filling

- 1 (8-oz) package cream cheese, softened
- 3 1/2 cups cold milk
- 2 (4-oz) packages instant chocolate pudding mix

Topping

- 1 (8-oz) package frozen whipped cream topping, thawed
- 1/4 cup topping with milk chocolate flavor
- 1/4 cup caramel filling
- 1/3 cup almond flakes

Direction:

1. Set oven to 200 degrees C (400 degrees F). Grease a 9 x 13-inch baking dish.

2. Melt the butter in the water in a medium-sized pan over medium heat. Pour the flour in one go and mix vigorously until the mixture forms a ball. Remove from heat and let stand for 5 minutes. Beat the eggs one by one until they are smooth and shiny. Spread in the prepared pan.

3. Bake in the preheated oven for 30 to 35 minutes, until puffed and browned. Cool completely on a rack.

4. While the puff pastry cools, mix the cream cheese mixture, the milk, and the pudding. Spread over the cooled puff pastry. Cool for 20 minutes.

5. Spread whipped cream on cooled topping and sprinkle with chocolate and caramel sauce. Sprinkle with almonds. Freeze 1 hour before serving.

Nutrition:

355 calories

22.3g fat

8.7g protein

3.5g Carbohydrates

11. Fresh Peach Dessert

Difficulty: Novice level

Preparation Time: 30 minutes

Cooking Time: 27 minutes

Servings: 15

Size/ portion: 1 cup

Ingredients

- 16 whole graham crackers, crushed
- 3/4 cup melted butter
- 1/2 cup white sugar
- 4 1/2 cups of miniature marshmallows
- 1/4 cup of milk
- 1 pint of heavy cream
- 1/3 cup of white sugar
- 6 large fresh peaches - peeled, seeded and sliced

Direction:

1. In a bowl, mix the crumbs from the graham cracker, melted butter, and 1/2 cup of sugar. Mix until a homogeneous mixture is obtained, save 1/4 cup of the mixture for filling. Squeeze the rest of the mixture into the bottom of a 9 x 13-inch baking dish.

2. Heat marshmallows and milk in a large pan over low heat and stir until marshmallows are completely melted. Remove from heat and let cool.

3. Beat the cream in a large bowl until soft peaks occur. Beat 1/3 cup of sugar until the cream forms firm spikes. Add the whipped cream to the cooled marshmallow mixture.

4. Divide half of the cream mixture over the crust, place the peaches over the cream and divide the rest of the cream mixture over the peaches. Sprinkle the crumb mixture on the cream. Cool until ready to serve.

Nutrition:

366 calories

22.5g fat

1.9g protein

7.6g Carbohydrates

- Brown sugar, ½ tablespoon
- Butter, low fat and unsalted, ½ teaspoon, melted

Directions:

1. Preheat an oven tray at 350F.

2. Set the fruits on the tray, and top with the brown sugar, mixed with the butter, and bake for 5 minutes.

3. Transfer to a platter.

Nutrition:

279 Calories 5.9g Fat

2.2g Protein 4.3g Carbohydrates

19. After Meal Apples
Difficulty: Intermediate level

Preparation Time: 15 minutes

Cooking Time: 25 minutes

Servings: 2

Size/ Portion: 1 piece

Ingredients:

- Apple, 1 whole, cut into chunks
- Pineapple chunks, ½ cups
- Grapes, seedless, ½ cup
- Orange juice, ¼ cup
- Cinnamon, ¼ teaspoon

Directions:

1. Preheat the oven to 350F.

2. Add all the fruits to a baking dish.

3. Drizzle with the orange juice and sprinkle with cinnamon.

4. Bake for 25 minutes, and serve hot.

Nutrition:

124 Calories 3.2g Fat

0.8g Protein

4.1g Carbohydrates

20. Warm Nut Bites
Difficulty: Intermediate level

Preparation Time: 10 minutes

Cooking Time: 20 minutes

Servings: 2

Size/ Portion 2 bites

Ingredients:

- Honey, 4 tablespoons
- Almonds, 2 cups
- Almond oil, 1 tablespoon

Directions:

1. Layer the almonds, whole, on a baking sheet.

2. Bake for 15 minutes at 350F.

3. Turn half way, and roll the almonds in honey.

4. Serve.

Nutrition:

268 Calories 19.7g Fat

7.6g Protein8.9g Carbohydrates

21. Dipped Sprouts
Difficulty: Intermediate level

Preparation Time: 12 minutes

Cooking Time: 10 minutes

Servings: 2

Size/ portion: 4 ounces

Ingredients:

- Brussels sprouts, 16 ounces
- Honey, 4 tablespoons
- Raisins and nuts, crushed, 6 tablespoons

Directions:

1. Boil water in a pot.

2. Add sprouts, and cook for 10 minutes until soft.

3.   Glaze the sprouts in honey, and coat well. Add nuts and raisins.

Nutrition:

221 Calories 15.1g Fat

5.3g Protein 6.7g Carbohydrates

22.   Pecans and Cheese

Difficulty: Intermediate level

Preparation Time: 20 minutes

Cooking Time: 0 minutes

Servings: 2

Size/ Portion: 3 ounces

Ingredients:

- Cinnamon, ground, 1 teaspoon
- Feta cheese, 4 ounces
- Pecans, finely chopped, 2 ounces
- Honey, 2 tablespoons
- Rosemary, fresh, 2 sprigs, minced

Directions:

1.   Make small balls of the cheese.

2.   Crush the pecans and place them in a shallow bowl with the cinnamon.

3.   Roll the cheese in the pecans and cinnamon. 4.   Drizzle honey over the balls.

5.   Serve with rosemary on top.

Nutrition:

234 Calories 18.6g Fat

7.5g Protein7.4g Carbohydrates

23.   Hazelnut Cookies

Difficulty: Professional level

Preparation Time: 8 minutes

Cooking Time: 21 minutes

Servings: 5

Size/ portion: 2 cookies

Ingredients:

- 1 1/4 cups hazelnut meal

- 6 tbsp. flour
- 1 tbsp. brown sugar
- 2 tbsp. powdered sugar
- 1/2 tsp. kosher salt
- 1/2 lemon zest
- 1/2 lemon juice
- 1/2 tsp. vanilla
- 1/4 cup extra virgin olive oil

Directions:

1.   Heat the oven at 375 degrees F.

2.   Take a bowl, add the hazelnut meal, brown sugar, flour, half of the powdered sugar, lemon zest, and salt. Next, whisk it well.

3.   Whisk olive oil and vanilla.

4.   Once the dough is crumbly, shape them into cookies and line them on the baking sheet.

5.   Bake it until the edges are lightly brown, around 20 minutes.

6.   Take out on a cooling rack Let it sit to cool.

7.   Meanwhile, take a small bowl and add lemon juice, and the remaining powdered sugar.

8.   Drizzle the syrup over the cookies before serving.

Nutrition: 276 Calories 3.6g Protein

21.2g Fat 17.5g Carbohydrates

24.   Fruit Dessert Nachos

Difficulty: Professional level

Preparation Time: 9 minutes

Cooking Time: 13 minutes

Servings: 3

Size/ Portion: 2 pieces

Ingredients:

- 1 tbsp. sugar

Directions:

1. Place a large pot on medium heat.
2. Once the pot is hot, add the quinoa, 45 grams at a time.
3. Stir the quinoa occasionally, until you start hearing it pop.
4. Once the popping starts, stir continuously for a minute.
5. Once you see that the quinoa has popped, place it in a small bowl.
6. Set up a double boiler and melt your chocolate.
7. Take a large bowl and add the chocolate, peanut butter powder, vanilla, and quinoa.
8. Mix it well to combine.
9. Place a parchment paper on the baking sheet.
10. Spread the chocolate batter across, making it around half an inch thick.
11. Mix together water and peanut butter to make the drizzle, and then drizzle it over the chocolate.
12. Swirl it around with a fork.
13. Refrigerate for it to set, and then slice them into small bars.

Nutrition: 170 Calories 4g Protein

8g Fat 13g Carbohydrates

29. Almond Honey Ricotta Spread

Difficulty: Professional level

Preparation Time: 7 minutes

Cooking Time: 15 minutes

Servings: 3

Size/ Portion: 2 tablespoons

Ingredients:

- 1/2 cup whole milk ricotta
- orange zest
- 1/4 cup sliced almonds
- 1/8 tsp. almond extract
- 1/2 tsp. honey
- sliced peaches
- honey to drizzle

Directions:

1. Take a medium bowl, and combine almonds, almond extract and ricotta.
2. Once you have stirred it well, place it in a bowl to serve.
3. Sprinkle with sliced almonds and drizzle some honey on the ricotta.
4. Spread a tablespoon of the spread to your choice of bread, top it with some honey and sliced peaches.

Nutrition:

199 Calories

8.5g Protein

12g Fat

17g Carbohydrates

30. Apricot Energy Bites

Difficulty: Professional level

Preparation Time: 16 minutes

Cooking Time: 0 minute

Servings: 10

Size/ Portion: 2 balls

Ingredients:

- 1 cup unsalted raw cashew nuts
- 1/4 tsp. ground ginger
- 1/2 cup dried apricots
- 2 3/4 tbsp. shredded, unsweetened coconut
- 2 tbsp. chopped dates
- 1 tsp. orange zest
- 1 tsp. lemon zest
- 1/4 tsp. cinnamon
- salt to taste

Directions:

1. Grind apricots, coconut, dates and cashew nuts in a processor.

2. Pulse until all a crumbly mixture has formed.

3. Add the spices, salt and citrus zest in the mixture.

4. Pulse it again to mix well.

5. Process the batter on high till it sticks together.

6. Take a dish or a tray and line it with parchment paper.

7. Shape the balls in your palm, make around 20 balls.

8. Keep in the refrigerator. Serve as needed.

Nutrition:

102 Calories

2g Protein

6g Fat

5g Carbohydrates

CHAPTER 10:

Sauces and Dressings

1.   Lemon Sauce

Preparation Time: 15 minutes

Cooking Time: 15 minutes

Servings: 6

Size/ Portion: 0.3 g

Ingredients:

- 2/3 cup lime juice
- 3 tablespoon extra virgin olive oil
- 1/4 cup diced scallions
- 3 tablespoons fresh dill
- 1/4 cup shallots, minced
- 1 tablespoons crushed garlic
- 1/2 teaspoon black pepper, fresh ground

Directions:

1. If using canned limes, use lime juice. Combine with oil and lime juice, along with the herbs, in a mixing bowl.
2. Combine all ingredients in a sauce pan. Simmer over medium-high heat.
3. Pour the sauce over the fish and vegetables mixture.

Nutrition

229 Calories 20g Fat

3.5g Protein 12g Carbohydrates

2.   Zesty Sauce

Preparation Time: 10 minutes

Cooking Time: 10 minutes

Servings: 4

Size/ Portion: 0.3 g

Ingredients:

- 2 teaspoon crushed garlic

- 1 tablespoon cornstarch
- 1 teaspoon parsley flakes
- 2 tablespoon light mayonnaise
- 1/2 teaspoon oregano
- 1 tablespoon dill, chopped
- 1/2 teaspoon crushed red pepper flakes
- Juice 1/2 lemon
- Options:
- Stuffed with shrimp, crabmeat or make as it is
- Stir in 1/2 cup vegetables, such as cucumbers, sun-dried tomatoes or peppers

Directions:

Mix all ingredients. Refrigerate for 20 minutes to thicken.

Nutrition

260 Calories

17g Fat

3g Protein

15g Carbohydrates

3.   Croquettes

Preparation Time: 15 minutes

Cooking Time: 15 minutes

Servings: 6

Size/ Portion: 0.5 g

Ingredients:

- 1 cup bread, cubed
- 1 cup cauliflower, cubed
- 2 tbsp vegan mayonnaise
- 2 tbsp vegan cheese, grated
- 2 cups spinach 2 teaspoons paprika

- 1 teaspoon lemon juice
- 1/2 cup chopped walnuts
- Salt and pepper to taste

Directions:

1. Combine all the ingredients together. Mold into croquettes.
2. Dip the croquettes in batter and fry in oil until brown.

Nutrition

250 Calories

20g Fat

3g Protein

18g Carbohydrates

4.   Tangy Dressing

Preparation Time: 15 minutes

Cooking Time: 0 minutes

Servings: 8

Size/ Portion: 0.3 g

Ingredients:

- 1/4 cup vegetable oil
- 1/4 cup orange juice
- 2 tablespoons fresh lemon juice
- 2 cloves garlic
- 4 tablespoons veganaise
- 2 tablespoon balsamic vinegar

Directions:

Mix all ingredients in a bowl. Mix well to blend.

Nutrition

154 Calories

9g Fat

3g Protein

21g Carbohydrates

5.   Butter Dressing

Preparation Time: 15 minutes

Cooking Time: 0 minutes

Servings: 4

Size/ Portion: 0.4 g

Ingredients:

- 1/2 cup vegan butter
- 1/2 cup vegan mayonnaise
- 1/4 cup balsamic vinegar
- Juice 1/2 lime
- 1/2 teaspoon garlic powder
- Salt and pepper to taste

Directions:

Combine all ingredients. Mix well.

Nutrition

249 Calories

25g Fat

2g Protein

14g Carbohydrates

Conclusion

With the Mediterranean diet pattern, you will come closer to nature as the entire food concept depends on fresh produce. Mealtime, in these lands, is nothing short of a celebration. People, living in these parts have a tradition of eating together. It is time to nurture interpersonal relations as well.

It is the right time to get into the stride and do something that will not only improve your current state but will also gift you a healthy future. After all, there is no more significant wealth than the health of an individual.

The primary aim of the Mediterranean diet is to make a person fit from within. Eating these foods will not only help in enhancing the outer physical appearance but will bring out the healthy inner glow. People with cardiovascular issues, blood pressure, blood sugar, stress and anxiety, and stomach related ailments will be benefited from this dietary program. Additionally, it will also improve the development of brain cells and activities.

Keeping all these things in mind, it is safe to conclude that the Mediterranean diet will improve a person's immune system. Someone with a robust immune system will be able to resist diseases easily. Thus, your desire of leading a healthy, fulfilling and constructive life will be achieved successfully.

The goal was to provide a thorough look at this diet and all the advantages and disadvantages it can bring to your life. As always, when making dietary changes you should consult your physician first to ensure this is a healthy change for you to achieve your goals in regard to your individual health. With the Mediterranean diet, much research has proven it is the most efficient method to lose weight and improve your overall health.

With this book, wanted to provide a detailed look at the Mediterranean lifestyle and exactly what it entails. The more informed you are about this diet and exactly what you should and should not be eating, the greater your chances of success will be!

People love incorporating a Mediterranean diet lifestyle because of how user-friendly it is! There are no counting calories, decreasing your portion sizes, or counting your intake of macronutrients diligently all day. It's about learning what the diet entails and making those choices to fill your pantry and fridge with fresh, healthy ingredients that will promote better health. You will be cutting out the unhealthy things like processed foods, artificial sugars, refined grains, and soda from your diet which are known to cause blood sugar spikes and excess weight gains. Instead, you'll be shopping for ingredients rich in vitamins, minerals, good fats, and antioxidants that will improve your health! With a menu allowing whole grains, fish, seafood, fruit, vegetables, and even a glass of wine a day, the Mediterranean diet allows for such variety that you can't get sick of it!

As long as you do this and stick to the simple rules of a Mediterranean diet, you can attain all the benefits it offers. One of the major benefits of this diet is that it is perfectly sustainable in the long run, not to mention, it is mouth-watering and delicious.

Once you start implementing the various protocols of this diet, you will see a positive change in your overall health. Ensure that you are being patient with yourself and stick to your diet without making any excuses.

7-Day Summer Meal plan

Days	Breakfast	Lunch/Dinner	Snack/dessert
1	Baked Bean Fish Meal	Grilled Whole Sea Bass	Marinated Feta and Artichokes
2	Mushroom Cod Stew	Pan-Cooked Fish with Tomatoes	Tuna Croquettes
3	Spiced Swordfish	Fish Steamed in Parchment with Veggies	Smoked Salmon Crudités
4	Anchovy Pasta Mania	Swordfish Souvlaki	Citrus-Marinated Olives
5	Shrimp Garlic Pasta	Stuffed Monkfish	Olive Tapenade with Anchovies
6	Vinegar Honeyed Salmon	Shrimp Santorini	Greek Deviled Eggs
7	Orange Fish Meal	Greek-Style Shrimp Cocktail	Manchego Crackers

7-Day Winter Meal plan

Days	Breakfast	Lunch/Dinner	Snack/dessert
1	Greek Stuffed Collard Greens	Rice with Vermicelli	Zucchini-Ricotta Fritters with Lemon-Garlic Aioli
2	Walnut Pesto Zoodles	Fava Beans and Rice	Salmon-Stuffed Cucumbers
3	Cauliflower Steaks with Eggplant Relish	Buttered Fava Beans	Sfougato
4	Mediterranean Lentil Sloppy Joes	Freekeh	Goat Cheese–Mackerel Pâté
5	Gorgonzola Sweet Potato Burgers	Fried Rice Balls with Tomato Sauce	Baba Ghanoush
6	Zucchini-Eggplant Gratin	Spanish-Style Rice	Instant Pot® Salsa
7	Grilled Stuffed Portobello Mushrooms	Zucchini with Rice and Tzatziki	Taste of the Mediterranean Fat Bombs

7-Day Autumn Meal Plan

Days	Breakfast	Lunch/Dinner	Snack/dessert
1	Watermelon Salad	Lemony Trout with Caramelized Shallots	Tuscan Kale Salad with Anchovies
2	Orange Celery Salad	Easy Tomato Tuna Melts	Roasted Garlic Hummus
3	Roasted Broccoli Salad	Mackerel and Green Bean Salad	Classic Hummus
4	Tomato Salad	Hazelnut Crusted Sea Bass	Tuscan Kale Salad with Anchovies
5	Feta Beet Salad	Shrimp and Pea Paella	Passion Fruit and Spicy Couscous
6	Cauliflower & Tomato Salad	Garlic Shrimp with Arugula Pesto	Spring Sandwich
7	Tahini Spinach	Baked Oysters with Vegetables	Springtime Quinoa Salad

7-Day Spring Meal Plan

Days	Breakfast	Lunch/Dinner	Snack/Dessert
1	Chicken Bruschetta Burgers	Baked Cod with Vegetables	Tomato Poached Fish with Herbs and Chickpeas
2	Chicken Cacciatore	Slow Cooker Salmon in Foil	Garlic Prawn and Pea Risotto
3	Chicken Gyros with Tzatziki Sauce	Dill Chutney Salmon	Honey and Vanilla Custard Cups with Crunchy Filo Pastry
4	Crispy Pesto Chicken	Garlic-Butter Parmesan Salmon and Asparagus	Mediterranean Tostadas
5	Beef Stew with Beans and Zucchini	Lemon Rosemary Roasted Branzino	Vegetable Ratatouille
6	Greek Beef Kebabs	Grilled Lemon Pesto Salmon	Citrus Cups
7	Chermoula Roasted Pork Tenderloin	Steamed Trout with Lemon Herb Crust	Mixed Berry Pancakes and Ricotta

Measurement Conversions

Volume Equivalents (Liquid)

US STANDARD	US STANDARD (OUNCES)	METRIC (APPROXIMATE)
2 tablespoons	1 fl. g	30 mL
¼ cup	2 fl. g	60 mL
½ cup	4 fl. g	120 mL
1 cup	8 fl. g	240 mL
1½ cups	12 fl. g	355 mL
2 cups or 1 pint	16 fl. g	475 mL
4 cups or 1 quart	32 fl. g	1 L
1 gallon	128 fl. g	4 L

Volume Equivalents (Dry)

US STANDARD	METRIC (APPROXIMATE)
1/8 teaspoon	0.5 mL
¼ teaspoon	1 mL
½ teaspoon	2 mL
¾ teaspoon	4 mL
1 teaspoon	5 mL
1 tablespoon	15 mL
¼ cup	59 mL
⅓ cup	79 mL
½ cup	118 mL
⅔ cup	156 mL
¾ cup	177 mL
1 cup	235 mL
2 cups or 1 pint	475 mL
3 cups	700 mL
4 cups or 1 quart	1 L

Oven Temperatures

FAHRENHEIT (F)	CELSIUS (C) (APPROXIMATE)
250°	120°
300°	150°
325°	165°
350°	180°
375°	190°
400°	200°
425°	220°
450°	230°

Weight Equivalents

US STANDARD	METRIC (APPROXIMATE)
½ ounce	15 g
1 ounce	30 g
2 ounces	60 g
4 ounces	115 g
8 ounces	225 g
12 ounces	340 g
16 ounces or 1 pound	455 g

References

American Heart Association. "American Heart Association Recommendations for Physical Activity in Adults." Accessed May 19, 2017. www.heart.org/HEARTORG/HealthyLiving/PhysicalActivity/FitnessBasics/American-Heart-Association-Recommendations-for-Physical-Activity-in-Adults_UCM_307976_Article.jsp#.WROL2kr3arV.

American Heart Association. "Mediterranean Diet with Virgin Olive Oil May Be Recipe for 'Good' Cholesterol." Accessed May 19, 2017. news.heart.org/mediterranean-diet-with-virgin-olive-oil-may-be-recipe-for-good-cholesterol.

American Heart Association. "Mediterranean-Style Diet Details." Accessed May 19, 2017. www.heart.org/HEARTORG/Affiliate/Mediterranean-style-diet-details_UCM_461758_Article.jsp#.WROPbUr3arU.

BMI Calculator. "Harris Benedict Equation." Accessed May 19, 2017. www.bmi-calculator.net/bmr-calculator/harris-benedict-equation.

Centers for Disease Control and Prevention. "Overweight & Obesity." Accessed May 19, 2017. www.cdc.gov/obesity.

Consumer Health Digest. "7 Healthiest Weight Loss Drinks That Really Work." Accessed May 19, 2017. www.consumerhealthdigest.com/weight-loss/7-healthiest-weight-loss-drinks.html.

Godman, Heidi. "Adopt a Mediterranean Diet Now for Better Health Later." Harvard Health Blog. Accessed May 19, 2017. www.health.harvard.edu/blog/adopt-a-mediterranean-diet-now-for-better-health-later-201311066846.

Gunnars, Kris, BSc. "5 Studies on the Mediterranean Diet—Does It Really Work?" Authority Nutrition. Accessed May 19, 2017. authoritynutrition.com/5-studies-on-the-mediterranean-diet.

Johns Hopkins Water Institute. "Water and Health." Accessed May 19, 2017. water.jhu.edu/index.php/about/water-health.

Mayo Clinic. "Mediterranean Diet: A Heart-Healthy Eating Plan." Accessed May 19, 2017. www.mayoclinic.org/healthy-lifestyle/nutrition-and-healthy-eating/in-depth/mediterranean-diet/art-20047801.

Mayo Clinic. "Water: How Much Should You Drink Every Day?" Accessed May 19, 2017. www.mayoclinic.org/healthy-lifestyle/nutrition-and-healthy-eating/in-depth/water/art-20044256.

Medline Plus, U.S. National Library of Medicine. "Obesity." Accessed May 19, 2017. medlineplus.gov/obesity.html.

Miller, Sara G. "Will Staying Hydrated Help with Weight Loss?" Live Science. Accessed May 19, 2017. www.livescience.com/55360-water-intake-weight-obesity.html.

Mozes, Alan. "Obesity May Be Bad for the Brain, Too." *U.S. News & World Report*. Accessed May 19, 2017. health.usnews.com/health-care/articles/2016-08-10/obesity-may-be-bad-for-the-brain-too.

CPSIA information can be obtained
at www.ICGtesting.com
Printed in the USA
BVHW060737030221
599247BV00010B/1126